OXFORD ASSESS AND PROGRESS

Series Editors

Katharine Boursicot
Reader in Medical Education and Deputy Head of the Centre for Medical and Healthcare Education,
St George's, University of London

David Sales
Consultant in Medi~ ~~ssment

Also available and forthcoming in the Oxford Assess and Progress series

Clinical Medicine, Second Edition
Alex Liakos and Martin Hill

Clinical Specialties, Second Edition
Lucy Etheridge and Alex Bonner

Situational Judgement Test, Second Edition
David Metcalfe and Harveer Dev

Medical Sciences
Jade Chow and John Patterson

Emergency Medicine
Pawan Gupta

Psychiatry
Gil Myers and Melissa Gardner

OXFORD ASSESS AND PROGRESS

Clinical Surgery

Edited by

Neil Borley

Consultant General and Colorectal Surgeon,
Cheltenham General Hospital, Cheltenham, UK

Frank Smith

Professor of Vascular Surgery and Surgical Education,
University of Bristol, Bristol, UK

Paul McGovern

ST5 Trauma and Orthopaedics,
South East Thames Rotation *and*
Clinical Teaching Fellow (Postgraduate),
UCL Medical School, London, UK

Bernadette Pereira

Specialty Registrar Trainee in General Surgery/Colorectal,
Royal Free Hospital NHS Trust, London, UK

Oliver Old

ST5 General Surgery,
Cheltenham General Hospital, Cheltenham, UK

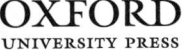

OXFORD
UNIVERSITY PRESS

OXFORD
UNIVERSITY PRESS

Great Clarendon Street, Oxford, OX2 6DP,
United Kingdom

Oxford University Press is a department of the University of Oxford.
It furthers the University's objective of excellence in research, scholarship,
and education by publishing worldwide. Oxford is a registered trade mark of
Oxford University Press in the UK and in certain other countries

Published in the United States of America by Oxford University Press
198 Madison Avenue, New York, NY 10016, United States of America

British Library Cataloguing in Publication Data

Data available

Library of Congress Control Number: 2013942164

ISBN 978–0–19–969642–0

Printed in Italy by
L.E.G.O. S.p.A.—Lavis TN

Series Editor Preface

The Oxford Assess and Progress Series is a groundbreaking development in the extensive area of self-assessment texts available for medical students. The questions were specifically commissioned for the series, written by practising clinicians, extensively peer-reviewed by students and their teachers, and quality assured to ensure that the material is up to date, accurate, and in line with modern testing formats.

The series has a number of unique features, and is designed to be as much a formative learning resource as a self-assessment one. The questions are constructed to test the same clinical problem-solving skills that we use as practising clinicians, rather than only to test theoretical knowledge. These skills include:

- gathering and using data required for clinical judgement
- choosing the appropriate examination and investigations, and interpretation of the findings
- applying knowledge
- demonstrating diagnostic skills
- ability to evaluate undifferentiated material
- ability to prioritize
- making decisions and demonstrating a structured approach to decision making.

Each question is bedded in reality and is typically presented as a clinical scenario, the content of which has been chosen to reflect the common and important conditions that most doctors are likely to encounter both during their training and in exams! The aim of the series is to build the reader's confidence in recognizing important symptoms and signs and suggesting the most appropriate investigations and management, and in so doing to aid the development of a clear approach to patient management which can be transferred to the wards.

The content of the series has deliberately been pinned to the relevant *Oxford Handbook*, but in addition has been guided by a blueprint which reflects the themes identified in *Tomorrow's Doctors* and *Good Medical Practice* to include novel areas such as history taking, recognition of signs (including red flags), and professionalism.

Particular attention has been paid to giving learning points and constructive feedback on each question, using clear fact- or evidence-based explanations as to why the correct response is right and why the incorrect responses are less appropriate. The question editorials are clearly referenced to the relevant sections of the accompanying *Oxford Handbook* and/or more widely to medical literature or guidelines. They are designed to guide and motivate the reader, being multi-purpose in nature and covering, for example, exam technique, approaches to difficult subjects, and links between subjects.

Another unique aspect of the series is the element of competency progression from being a relatively inexperienced student to being a more experienced junior doctor. We have suggested the following four degrees of difficulty to reflect the level of training, so that the reader can monitor their own progress over time:

- graduate should know★
- graduate nice to know★★
- foundation doctor should know★★★
- foundation doctor nice to know★★★

We advise the reader to attempt the questions in blocks as a way of testing their knowledge in a clinical context. The series can be treated as a dress rehearsal for life on the ward by using the material to hone clinical acumen and build confidence by encouraging a clear, consistent, and rational approach, proficiency in recognizing and evaluating symptoms and signs, making a rational differential diagnosis, and suggesting appropriate investigations and management.

Adopting such an approach can aid not only success in examinations, which really are designed to confirm learning, but also—more importantly—being a good doctor. In this way we can deliver high-quality and safe patient care by recognizing, understanding, and treating common problems, but at the same time remaining alert to the possibility of less likely but potentially catastrophic conditions.

Katharine Boursicot and David Sales, Series Editors

A Note on Single Best Answer and Extended Matching Questions

Single best answer questions are currently the format of choice being widely used by most undergraduate and postgraduate knowledge tests, and therefore most of the assessment questions in this book follow this format.

Briefly, the single best answer question presents a problem, usually a clinical scenario, before presenting the question itself and a list of five options. These consist of one correct answer and four incorrect options or 'distractors' from which the reader has to choose a response.

Extended matching questions, also known as extended matching items, were introduced as a more reliable way of testing knowledge. They are still widely used in many undergraduate and postgraduate knowledge tests, and are therefore included in this book.

An extended matching question is organized as one list of possible options followed by a set of items, usually clinical scenarios. The correct response to each item must be chosen from the list of options.

All of the questions in this book, which are typically based on an evaluation of symptoms, signs, or results of investigations either as single entities or in combination, are designed to test *reasoning* skills rather than straightforward recall of facts, and utilize cognitive processes similar to those used in clinical practice.

The peer-reviewed questions are written and edited in accordance with contemporary best assessment practice, and their content has been guided by a blueprint pinned to all areas of *Good Medical Practice*, which ensures comprehensive coverage.

The answers and their rationales are evidence-based and have been reviewed to ensure that they are absolutely correct. Incorrect options are selected as being plausible, and indeed they may appear correct to the less knowledgeable reader. When answering questions, the reader may wish to use the 'cover' test in which they read the scenario and the question but cover the options.

Katharine Boursicot and David Sales, Series Editors

Acknowledgements

Figure 5.3 reproduced from Mason, G. 'Management of the patient with inflammatory breast cancer,' *ONCOLOGY Nurse Edition,* 22:8, 2008, with permission from UBM Media.

Contents

About the Editors

Volume editors

Neil Borley is a Consultant Colorectal Surgeon at Cheltenham General Hospital with a wide experience of undergraduate and postgraduate teaching including being Clinical Tutor in Surgery for the Clinical School in Oxford. He has been/is an examiner both for Medical Finals and Postgraduate qualifications in surgery and has written or edited numerous textbooks particularly at undergraduate level.

Frank Smith is Professor of Vascular Surgery and Surgical Education at the University of Bristol. He has significant commitments to both undergraduate and postgraduate education and has been an external examiner in undergraduate education to several medical schools. He is a member of the Court of Examiners of the Royal College of Surgeons of England and Chair of Quality Assurance for the UEMS Fellowship of the European Boards of Vascular Surgery (FEBVS) examinations.

Paul McGovern is an Orthopaedic Registrar in London and Clinical Teaching Fellow in Postgraduate Medical Education at UCL Medical School. He is an examiner for MBBS finals and writes examination questions for the General Medical Council's Fitness to Practice programme.

Bernadette Pereira is a Specialty Registrar in General Surgery on the London Deanery Higher Surgical Training Programme. She is a keen Medical Educator, having done a Post Graduate Certificate in Medical Education, OSCE examiner, MCQ/EMQ/SBA writer for UCL exam question bank, and was a PLAB associate for the General Medical Council.

Oliver Old is a Specialist Registrar in General Surgery, having completed Basic Surgical Training in Severn Deanery, and Higher Surgical Training in Severn and Peninsula Deaneries. He has experience of undergraduate and postgraduate teaching.

Series editors

Katharine Boursicot is a reader in Medical Education and Deputy Head of the Centre for Medical and Healthcare Education at St George's, University of London. Previously she was Head of Assessment at Barts and The London, and Associate Dean for Assessment for Cambridge University School of Medicine. She is consultant on assessment to several UK medical schools, Royal Colleges, and international institutions as well as General Medical Council PLAB Part 2 Panel and Fitness to Practise clinical skills testing.

David Sales is a general practitioner by training who has been involved in medical assessment for over 20 years, having previously been convenor of the MRCGP knowledge test. He has run item writing workshops for a number of undergraduate medical schools, medical Royal Colleges, and internationally. For the General Medical Council he currently chairs the Professional and Linguistic Assessment Boards Part 1 panel and is their consultant on Fitness to Practise knowledge testing.

Contributors

Asmaa Al-Alaak
ST5 Breast Surgery
Gloucestershire Hospitals, UK

Neil Borley
Consultant General and
Colorectal Surgeon
Cheltenham General Hospital
Cheltenham, UK

Olivier Branford
Extremity Reconstruction Fellow
ST8 Plastic Surgery
Imperial College Healthcare
NHS Trust
London, UK

Gemma Conn
Consultant Colorectal Surgeon
Broomfield Hospital
Chelmsford, UK

Sebastian Dawson-Bowling
Consultant Orthopaedic Surgeon
Barts Health NHS Trust
London, UK

Simon Fisher
ST8 Liver Surgery & Transplant
Queen Elizabeth Hospital
Birmingham, UK

Serena Ledwidge
Consultant Oncoplastic Breast
Surgeon
St Bartholomew's Hospital
London, UK

Paul McGovern
ST5 Trauma and Orthopaedics
South East Thames Rotation *and*
Clinical Teaching Fellow
(Postgraduate)
UCL Medical School
London, UK

Oliver Old
ST5 General Surgery
Cheltenham General Hospital
Cheltenham, UK

Bernadette Pereira
Specialty Registrar Trainee in
General Surgery/Colorectal
Royal Free Hospital NHS Trust
London, UK

Frank Smith
Professor of Vascular Surgery and
Surgical Education
University of Bristol
Bristol, UK

James Wood
ST5 Colorectal Surgery
Gloucestershire Hospitals, UK

Normal and Average Values

	Normal value
Haematology	
White cell count (WCC)	4–11 × 10⁹/L
Haemoglobin (Hb)	M: 13.5–18g/dL F: 11.5–16g/dL
Packed cell volume (PCV)	M: 0.4–0.54L/L F: 0.37–0.47L/L
Mean corpuscular volume (MCV)	76–96fL
Neutrophils	2–7.5 × 10⁹/L
Lymphocytes	1.3–3.5 × 10⁹/L
Eosinophils	0.04–0.44 × 10⁹/L
Basophils	0–0.1 × 10⁹/L
Monocytes	0.2–0.8 × 10⁹/L
Platelets	150–400 × 10⁹/L
Reticulocytes	25–100 × 10⁹/L
Erythrocyte sedimentation rate (ESR)	<20mm/h (but age dependent; see → OHCM p356)
Prothrombin time (PT)	10–14s
Activated partial thromboplastin time (aPTT)	35–45s
International normalized ratio (INR)	0.9–1.2
Biochemistry	
Alanine aminotransferase (ALT)	5–35IU/L
Albumin	35–50g/L
Alkaline phosphatase (ALP)	30–150U/L
Amylase	0–180U/dL
Aspartate transaminase (AST)	5–35IU/L
Bilirubin	3–17μmol/L
Calcium (total)	2.12–2.65mmol/L
Chloride	95–105mmol/L
Cortisol	450–750nmol/L (am) 80–280nmol/L (midnight)
C-reactive protein (CRP)	<10mg/L

Creatine kinase	M: 25–195IU/L F: 25–170IU/L
Creatinine	70–<150µmol/L
Ferritin	12–200mcg/L
Folate	3–16micrograms/L
Gamma-glutamyl transpeptidase (GGT)	M: 11–51IU/L F: 7–33IU/L
Lactate dehydrogenase (LDH)	70–250IU/L
Magnesium	0.75–1.05mmol/L
Osmolality	278–305mOsmol/kg
Potassium	3.5–5mmol/L
Protein (total)	60–80g/L
Sodium	135–145mmol/L
Thyroid stimulating hormone (TSH)	0.5–5.7mu/L
Thyroxine (T_4)	70–140nmol/L
Thyroxine (free)	9–22pmol/L
Urate	M: 210–480mmol/L F: 150–390mmol/L
Urea	2.5–6.7mmol/L
Vitamin B_{12}	0.13–0.68mmol/L
Arterial blood gases	
pH	7.35–7.45
PaO_2	>10.6kPa
$PaCO_2$	4.7–6.0kPa
Base excess	±2mmol/L
Urine	
Cortisol (free)	<280nmol/24h
Osmolality	350–1000mOsmol/kg
Potassium	14–120mmol/24h
Protein	<150mg/24h
Sodium	100–250mmol/24h

Abbreviations

AFP	alpha-fetoprotein
ASA	American Society of Anesthesiologists
ATLS	advanced trauma life support
BMI	body mass index
bpm	beats per minute
CABG	coronary artery bypass grafting
CRP	C-reactive protein
ELISA	enzyme-linked immunosorbent assay
ENT	ear, nose, and throat
ERCP	endoscopic retrograde cholangiopancreatography
FBC	full blood count
FNAB	fine-needle aspiration biopsy
FSH	follicle-stimulating hormone
GCS	Glasgow Coma Scale
GI	gastrointestinal
GP	general practitioner
HCG	human chorionic gonadotrophin
IV	intravenous
KUB	kidneys, ureter, bladder
LDH	lactate dehydrogenase
LFT	liver function test
MRCP	magnetic resonance cholangiopancreatography
MRI	magnetic resonance imaging
NICE	National Institute for Health and Clinical Excellence
NSAID	non-steroidal anti-inflammatory drug
NSGCT	non-seminomatous germ cell tumour
OGD	oesophagogastroduodenoscopy
PO	orally
SC	subcutaneous
T_3	tri-iodothyronine
T_4	thyroxine
TED	thromboembolus deterrent
TSH	thyroid stimulating hormone
U&E	urea and electrolytes
VTE	venous thromboembolism

How to Use this Book

Oxford Assess and Progress, Surgery has been carefully designed to ensure you get the most out of your revision and are prepared for your exams. Here is a brief guide to some of the features and learning tools.

Organization of content

Chapter editorials will help you unpick tricky subjects, and when it's late at night and you need something to remind you why you're doing this, you'll find words of encouragement!

Chapters begin with **Single Best Answer (SBAs)** questions followed by **Extended Matching Questions (EMQs)** questions. Answers can be found at the end of each chapter beginning with the SBA answers, and then the EMQ answers.

How to read an answer

Unlike other revision guides on the market, this one is crammed full of feedback, so you should understand exactly why each answer is correct, and gain an insight into the common pitfalls. With every answer there is an explanation of why that particular choice is the most appropriate. For some questions there is additional explanation of why the distractors are less suitable. Where relevant you will also be directed to sources of further information, such as the *Oxford Handbook of Clinical Surgery*, websites, and journal articles.

→ http://www.nice.org.uk/nicemedia/pdf/word/CG43NICEGuide line.doc

Progression points

The questions in every chapter are ordered by level of difficulty and competence, indicated by the following symbols:

★   *Graduate 'should know'*—you should be aiming to get most of these correct.

★★   *Graduate 'nice to know'*—these are a bit tougher but not above your capabilities.

★★★   *Foundation Doctor 'should know'*—these will really test your understanding.

★★★★ *Foundation Doctor 'nice to know'*—give these a go when you're ready to challenge yourself.

Oxford Handbook of Clinical Surgery

The *Oxford Handbook of Clinical Surgery* page references are given with the answers to some questions, e.g. OH Clin Surg, 4th edn → p402. Please note that this reference is the 4th edition of the *Oxford Handbook of Clinical Surgery*, and that other editions are unlikely to have the same material in exactly the same place.

Chapter 1

Principles of surgery

Asmaa Al-Alaak

Modern surgery is possibly the most complete discipline in medicine today. It combines the need for understanding of the complete range of pathological processes that befall the human body from neoplasia and microbiological disease to degenerative and genetic related conditions. There is a need to be familiar with the latest concepts in how to monitor and manage the physiological processes of the body whilst still needing to understand when and how treatment, surgical and non-surgical, should be used. The modern student or trainee must be able to master all these disciplines. Integrating the understanding of basic body processes with the principles of how and when to support, prevent, or replace them forms the core of the principles of surgery. In the following sections, the questions will cover all these principles.

This first chapter also covers the key points of the assessment of surgical disease by history and examination as well as how pathological processes in organ systems can affect patients coming to surgery. Lastly, every doctor needs to understand the basic facts about how surgical operations and procedures are conducted and how patients are kept safe during surgery.

Neil Borley

QUESTIONS

Single Best Answers

1. A 65-year-old man has been diagnosed with cancer of the colon and requires a right hemicolectomy. He is not undergoing preoperative bowel preparation. He is a non-insulin-dependent diabetic currently on gliclazide modified release 60mg and metformin 500mg. The patient requires a prescription for his diabetic control for the day before surgery. Which is the *single* most appropriate first line of management in addition to monitoring his blood glucose? ★

A Give normal dose of metformin and gliclazide

B Omit both metformin and gliclazide

C Omit gliclazide and give normal dose of metformin

D Omit metformin and give normal dose of gliclazide

E Start IV insulin regimen—sliding scale

2. A 70-year-old woman has a proximal ileostomy following emergency surgery for small bowel obstruction. This has resulted in high-output fluid losses from the stoma. In order to maintain her nutritional status she is commenced on central total parenteral nutrition. During the first week of total parenteral nutrition the patient's bloods need to be monitored. Which is the *single* most appropriate group of investigations required? ★★

A Daily full blood count (FBC), urea and electrolytes (U&E)

B Daily FBC, U&E, and liver function tests (LFTs)

C Daily U&E, LFTs, and glucose

D Daily U&E, LFTs, and micronutrients

E Daily U&E and glucose, twice weekly LFTs, weekly micronutrients

3. A 25-year-old man who has had no other health problems has been troubled by a discharging pilonidal sinus over the last 2 years. Arrangements have been made for him to undergo excision of this sinus under general anaesthetic as a day case procedure. Which is the *single* most appropriate option for his thromboprophylaxis? ★★★

A None

B Thromboembolus deterrent (TED) stockings only

C TED stockings and 2500IU of low-molecular-weight heparin SC once a day

D TED stockings and 5000IU of low-molecular-weight heparin SC once a day

E 2500IU of low-molecular-weight heparin SC once a day

4. A 30-year-old woman presents with 2 days of central abdominal pain radiating to the right iliac fossa. Following clinical assessment a diagnosis of appendicitis is made. She undergoes a laparoscopic appendicectomy and at the time it is noted that the appendix was inflamed but not perforated. Which is the *single* most appropriate choice of antibiotic prophylaxis? ★

A Gentamicin 120mg IV—single dose at induction

B Flucloxacillin 1g IV + gentamicin 120mg IV + amoxicillin 500mg IV—single dose at induction

C Flucloxacillin 1g IV + gentamicin 120mg IV + amoxicillin 500mg IV—at induction and 5 days post-op

D Gentamicin 120mg IV + metronidazole 500mg IV + amoxicillin 500 mg IV—single dose at induction

E Gentamicin 120mg IV + metronidazole 500mg IV + amoxicillin 500 mg IV—at induction and for 5 days post-op

5. An 80-year-old man is admitted as an emergency with abdominal pain. He suffers from dementia and lives in a nursing home. Unfortunately there is no available information on his current condition and past medical history. On examination he has a single stoma sited in the right iliac fossa as shown in Figure 1.1 which is producing thick green-brown material.

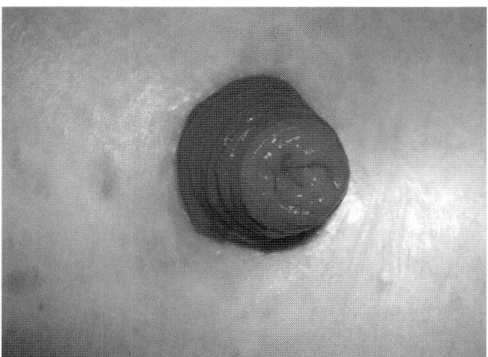

Figure 1.1 Stoma sited in the right iliac fossa

Which is the *single* most likely type of stoma present? ★★

A End colostomy

B End jejunostomy

C End ileostomy

D Loop ileostomy

E Urostomy

6. A 60-year-old woman is 1 day following hip replacement surgery and has been prescribed 3 units of blood for an elective transfusion. The nurse looking after the patient is concerned that halfway through the first unit of blood the patient started complaining of back pain. Her blood pressure has dropped from 125/95mmHg to 70/50mmHg, her pulse is 120bpm, temperature is 39°C, and her respiratory rate is 25 breaths per min. Which is the *single* most appropriate first step in the management of this patient? ★

A Administer 3L/min oxygen via non-rebreathing mask/bag

B Give 500mL 0.9% saline IV immediately

C Start empirical broad-spectrum antibiotics

D Stop transfusion immediately

E Take blood cultures

7. A 66-year-old man is 10 days following a right axillary-femoral bypass graft for occlusive peripheral vascular disease. The patient has developed a large pulsatile swelling in his right groin with blood oozing from the surgical scar over the last 20min. Which is the *single* most appropriate next step in the management of this patient? ★★★

A Administer 2500IU heparin

B Apply a compression dressing and review in 30min

C Arrange an urgent angiogram

D Check clotting studies and FBC

E Get senior help

8. A 47-year-old woman is admitted as an emergency with severe acute pancreatitis. As part of her clinical management she has a urinary catheter. Over the last 6h her urine output has been 20, 10, 0, 7, 0, 0mL/h drained. Blood pressure is 120/85mmHg and pulse 82bpm (both unchanged over the last 6h). Which is the *single* most appropriate next step in the management of this patient? ★★★

A Check urinary catheter is not blocked by flushing

B Give 500mL of IV 0.9% saline over 2h

C Give 40mg furosemide IV stat

D Insert central venous pressure line

E Observe patient

9. A 72-year-old man has undergone a rigid cystoscopy under the care of the urologists. He has been recommenced on warfarin which he takes for atrial fibrillation. His international normalized ratio comes back as >5.0. He has had no postoperative bleeding and is clinically well. Which is the *single* most appropriate next step in the treatment of this patient? ★★★

A Give 1mg vitamin K IV stat

B Give 10mg vitamin K IV stat

C Give fresh frozen plasma 1 unit IV over 2h

D Give fresh frozen plasma 1 unit IV over 2h and 5mg vitamin K IM stat

E Omit next dose of warfarin

10. A 35-year-old woman is seen in pre-admission clinic a week before she is scheduled for bilateral varicose vein surgery. She is a fit lady with no past medical history and is currently taking an oestrogen-only oral contraceptive pill. Which is the *single* most appropriate description of the advice she should be given? ★★

A Advise patient to continue the oestrogen-only oral contraceptive pill

B Advise patient to stop the oestrogen-only oral contraceptive pill

C Advise patient to see GP

D Advise patient to switch to a progesterone-only pill

E Inform a senior member of the team

11. An 80-year-old man has undergone emergency surgery for intestinal obstruction due to an obstructed hernia. Two days following surgery he has been vomiting despite his nasogastric tube and has developed a temperature of 38°C, he feels short of breath, and his pulse is 120bpm. On auscultation of his chest there is reduced air entry and coarse crackles on the right lung base. A chest X-ray is taken and shown in Figure 1.2.

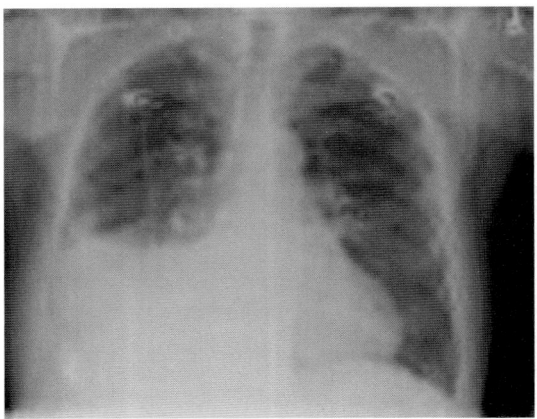

Figure 1.2 The chest X-ray taken

Which is the *single* most likely diagnosis? ★

A Acute respiratory distress syndrome

B Aspiration pneumonia

C Atelectasis

D Pulmonary embolus

E Pulmonary oedema

12. A 45-year-old man is admitted as a day case for arthroscopy of the right knee. He has a past medical history of asthma which is usually well controlled with inhalers. Which is the *single* best grade to describe his co-morbidity according to the American Society of Anesthesiologists (ASA) system? ★

A ASA I

B ASA II

C ASA III

D ASA IV

E ASA V

13. A 33-year-old woman has been admitted as an emergency with abdominal pain. She suffers from epilepsy and has been on anti-convulsant medication for a number of years. As part of her initial management she was kept nil by mouth pending further investigation and has had no anticonvulsant therapy for 2 days as a result. She has suffered a series of fits without regaining consciousness. Which is the *single* most appropriate first step in the management of this patient? ★★

A Administer high-flow oxygen

B Administer diazepam 10mg IV

C Check blood glucose

D Clear the oral cavity and insert an airway support

E Start a phenytoin infusion

14. A 27-year-old man is admitted to hospital following an industrial accident. He has sustained 30% by surface area partial thickness burns. The burns have been treated conservatively with dressings. A week into his hospital stay it is noted that he has a blue/green discharge from one of the wounds with a sweet odour. Which is the *single* most likely causative organism? ★★

A *Escherichia coli*

B *Proteus mirabilis*

C *Pseudomonas aeruginosa*

D *Staphylococcus aureus*

E *Streptococcus pyogenes*

15. A 67-year-old man is recovering in hospital following surgery for carcinoma of the colon. He has no past medical history and takes no regular medications. Five days following surgery his pulse rate has gone rapidly up to 150bpm and is irregular. His blood pressure has fallen directly from 135/80mmHg to 80/45mmHg. An urgent electro-cardiogram (ECG) is performed as shown in Figure 1.3.

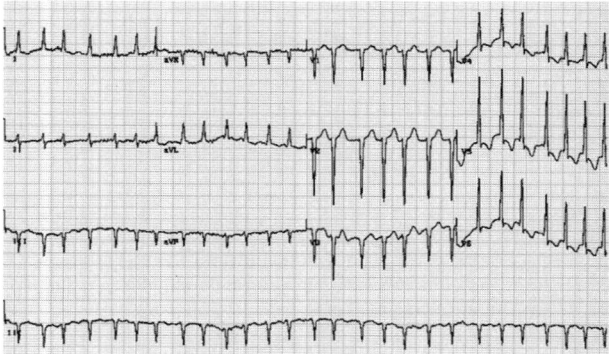

Figure 1.3 An urgent ECG is performed

Which is the *single* most appropriate next step in the management of this patient? ★★★

A Administer propranolol 40mg PO stat

B Arrange for DC cardioversion

C Administer digoxin 125mcg PO stat

D Arrange a computed tomography (CT) scan of the abdomen and pelvis

E Give IV metronidazole 500mg IV and gentamicin 120mg IV stat

16. A 57-year-old man is admitted via the emergency department with an umbilical hernia. He is known to suffer from liver cirrhosis secondary to high alcohol use. He has an irreducible and tender umbilical hernia which requires urgent surgical intervention. After completion of his clinical assessment he is found to fall into Child's A classification of surgical risk. Which is the *single* most likely clinical finding in this patient? ★★★

A Extensive ascites

B Good nutritional status

C Moderate neurological dysfunction

D Serum albumin 25g/L

E Serum bilirubin <20mg/L

17. A 24-year-old man has sustained a deep laceration to the palm of the hand with evidence of a tendon injury. Neurological examination of the arm is normal. He undergoes exploration and repair with the assistance of a tourniquet placed around the arm to reduce intraoperative bleeding. A few days following his surgery he has numbness on the dorsal aspect of his hand affecting the medial three digits and medial half of the index finger. Which is the *single* most likely nerve to have been injured during surgery by tourniquet pressure? ★★★★

A Lateral cutaneous nerve of the forearm

B Median nerve

C Musculocutaneous nerve

D Radial nerve

E Ulnar nerve

18. A 70-year-old woman has a longstanding foot ulcer due to peripheral vascular disease. There is large deep ulcer on the medial aspect of her right lower leg with cellulitis extending towards the knee. She has a temperature of 38°C and pulse of 100bpm. She is started on IV flucloxacillin and benzylpenicillin. Ten days later she develops lower abdominal pain and offensive green diarrhoea. Which is the *single* most likely causative organism? ★★

A *Escherichia coli*

B *Campylobacter jejuni*

C *Clostridium difficile*

D *Salmonella typhi*

E *Shigella sonnei*

19. A 85-year-old man is admitted following a fall at home. He has chronic obstructive pulmonary disease for which he requires regular nebulizers and occasional oxygen at home. He has a fractured neck of the right femur for which he undergoes surgery. Two days following the procedure he becomes increasingly severely short of breath on the high dependency unit despite supplemental oxygen, IV fluids, and physiotherapy. Pulse oximetry shows an oxygen saturation of 80%. Arterial blood gas results are pH 7.25, PaO_2 5kPa, $PaCO_2$ 8kPa, and bicarbonate of 30mmol/L. Which is the *single* most appropriate next step in his management? ★★★★

A Biphasic positive pressure ventilation (BiPAP)

B Continuous positive airway pressure (CPAP)

C Intermittent positive pressure ventilation (IPPV)

D Oxygen administration via high-flow (Venturi) face mask

E Oxygen administration via low-flow (Hudson) face mask

20. A 26-year-old woman is admitted with 2 days of lower abdominal pain associated with vomiting. A diagnosis of possible viral gastroenteritis is made. She is kept nil by mouth. The following day her serum potassium is 6.3mmol/L. Which is the *single* most appropriate next step in the management of this patient? ★★★

A Consider haemodialysis

B Give 10mL calcium gluconate 10% IV stat

C Give 50mL 50% dextrose with 15 units of actrapid stat

D Give calcium resonium 30g enema

E Repeat U&E and perform an ECG

21. A 40-year-old woman is admitted as a day case for excision of a lipoma under local anaesthetic. She has no past medical history, is not on any medications, and is not known to have any allergies. Shortly after starting the procedure the patient suddenly starts complaining of light-headedness, numbness of her tongue, and her speech becomes slurred. Which is the *single* most likely diagnosis? ★★

A Cerebrovascular event ('stroke')

B Drug-induced anaphylaxis

C Epileptic seizure

D Local anaesthetic toxicity

E Vasovagal syncope

22. An 85-year-old woman is admitted to hospital following a fall. A chest X-ray demonstrates bilateral pneumothoraces and bilateral chest drains are inserted in the emergency department. The following day the left-sided chest drain has stopped swinging and there is evidence of neck swelling with subcutaneous crepitus. Which is the *single* most likely diagnosis? ★

A Empyema

B Haemothorax

C Pleural effusion

D Pulmonary oedema

E Surgical emphysema

23. A 70-year-old woman is admitted to hospital with complications of a pharyngeal pouch and chronically poor nutrition. A fine-bore feeding tube has just been inserted for enteral nutrition on the ward. Which is the *single* most appropriate next step in the management of this patient prior to use of the tube? ★

A Assess pH of nasogastric aspirate

B Auscultate over the upper abdomen during air injection into the tube

C Perform a contrast X-ray of the nasogastric tube

D Request a chest X-ray

E Perform a trial injection of saline down the tube

24. A 53-year-old man is going to theatre for a laparoscopic cholecystectomy. The anaesthetist prescribes a dose of medication to be administered 1h prior to scheduled theatre time. Which is the *single* most likely prescription? ★

A Buscopan 10mg PO

B Chlorpheniramine 10mg PO

C Diazepam 10mg PO

D Midazolam 5mg IV

E Morphine 10mg PO

Extended Matching Questions

Scanning

For each scenario choose the *single* most appropriate next investigation from the list of options. Each option may be used once, more than once, or not at all.

A Abdominopelvic CT scan

B Colour flow Doppler (duplex) ultrasound scan

C Doppler ultrasound

D Endoanal ultrasound scan

E Pelvic magnetic resonance imaging (MRI) scan

F Transabdominal ultrasound scan

G Transduodenal endoscopic ultrasound scan

H Transrectal ultrasound scan

I Transvaginal ultrasound scan

1. A 65-year-old man with no symptoms is undergoing routine screening for the presence of abdominal aortic aneurysm. ★★★

2. A 25-year-old woman is admitted with 48h of lower abdominal and pelvic pain. A diagnosis of torted ovarian cyst is suspected. ★

3. A 27-year-old lady is suffering from anorectal incontinence following the delivery of her second child by emergency forceps 8 months ago. ★★★

4. A 57-year-old man presents with 9 months of intermittent right upper quadrant abdominal pain, radiating to the right side and subscapular region usually precipitated by food and associated with nausea. ★★

5. A 40-year-old woman is being assessed for the presence of saphenofemoral venous reflux as a cause for her varicose veins. ★

Respiratory distress

For each scenario choose the *single* most likely diagnosis from the list of options. Each option may be used once, more than once, or not at all.

A Acute lung injury

B Air embolus

C Atelectasis

D Acute respiratory distress syndrome

E Fat embolus

F Pneumonia

G Pneumothorax

H Pulmonary embolism

I Pulmonary oedema

J Pleural effusion

6. A 40-year-old man is recovering in hospital following an open chol-ecystectomy. He has no past medical history but he has been a smoker for most of his adult life. On day two after his surgery he spikes a temperature of 38°C, heart rate is 110bpm, and his oxygen saturation on air is 85%. He has reduced air entry bilaterally and his chest is dull to percussion. ★★

7. A 67-year-old woman is admitted to the emergency department following a fall. She has sustained a complex femoral shaft fracture. She has no past medical history and is not on any medications. Within 24h of surgery to repair the fracture she develops a temperature of 38.2°C, heart rate is 115bpm, respiratory rate is 25 breaths/min, and her Glasgow Coma Scale score is 12/15. She also has a generalized pete-chial rash. ★★

8. A 56-year-old man is admitted with rectal bleeding. He has a past medical history of diverticular disease but is otherwise fit and well with no other medical problems. He has a further bleed and his haemo-globin drops to 7.9. Within a few hours of starting a blood transfusion he suddenly becomes short of breath and hypoxic. On examination he has bilateral basal crackles. An ECG is normal. ★★

9. A 38-year-old woman is convalescing at home following major gynaecological surgery. She is admitted 2 weeks following her sur-gery with increasing shortness of breath. Heart rate is 105bpm, oxygen saturation 89% on air, and she has a tender right calf. ★

10. A 20-year-old IV drug user is admitted with swelling of his left groin and widespread cellulitis of the leg. He requires IV anti-biotics but peripheral access has not been possible; thus a central line is inserted in his neck. Following the procedure he becomes increasingly short of breath and hypoxic. On examination of his chest the right side is resonant to percussion and there is no air entry. ★

Decontamination methods

For each scenario choose the *single* most appropriate method of decontamination from the list of options. Each option may be used once, more than once, or not at all.

A Acetaldehyde solution (Cidex®)

B Aqueous gel solution of alcohol (Aquagel®)

C Cationic soap solution (chlorhexidine)

D Chloroxylenol solution (Dettol®)

E Ethyl alcohol (100%) swabs

F Gamma radiation

G Hydrogen peroxide solution

H Organic dye preparation (Proflavine®)

I Povidone-iodine alcoholic solution (Betadine®)

11. A 65-year-old woman with suspected perforated diverticulitis is going to theatre and requires a peripheral venous catheter insertion. As part of the procedure the skin must be prepared with antiseptic. ★

12. A 70-year-old man is scheduled to undergo a colonoscopy. The colonoscope must be disinfected prior to the procedure. ★★★

13. A 24-year-old woman is about to undergo laparoscopic appendicectomy and you are scrubbing in to assist with the procedure. ★★

14. A 40-year-old man has developed a chronic complex fistula in ano with multiple tracks in the perineum. He is going to theatre to have the fistula cleansed under anaesthetic. ★★

15. A 45-year-old woman is due to undergo an open hysterectomy for extensive fibroids. The abdominal skin surface needs to be prepared prior to surgical draping. ★★★

Acid–base disturbances

For each scenario choose the *single* most likely acid–base disturbance from the list of options. Each option may be used once, more than once, or not at all.

A Compensated metabolic acidosis

B Compensated metabolic alkalosis

C Compensated respiratory acidosis

D Compensated respiratory alkalosis

E Uncompensated metabolic acidosis

F Uncompensated metabolic alkalosis

G Uncompensated respiratory acidosis

H Uncompensated respiratory alkalosis

I Normal

16. A 90-year-old man is admitted to the emergency department suffering 1 day of severe abdominal pain. This is associated with abdominal distension and bloody diarrhoea. He has a past medical history of atrial fibrillation. He is hypotensive and tachycardic, his abdomen is distended and mildly tender. An arterial blood sample is taken and the results are: pH 7.2, PaO_2 9kPa, $PaCO_2$ 3.7kPa, HCO_3^- 18.7mmol/L, and a lactate of 7. ★★

17. An 80-year-old woman is admitted with a fractured neck of femur. She is given some morphine intravenously for pain control. Her respiratory rate drops to 8 breaths per minute. Her arterial blood gas results are: pH 7.25, PaO_2 7kPa, $PaCO_2$ 8kPa, HCO_3^- 23mmol/L. ★★

18. A 25-year-old woman is admitted with lower abdominal pain. She is a known asthmatic and soon after admission she becomes breathless and unable to complete full sentences. Her blood gas results are: pH 7.5, PaO_2 8kPa, $PaCO_2$ 3.7kPa, HCO_3^- 19mmol/L. ★★

19. A 44-year-old man with known alcohol addiction is admitted with a 2-day history of upper abdominal pain and vomiting. His amylase on admission is >2000IU/L. His blood gas results are: pH 7.35, PaO_2 12kPa, $PaCO_2$ 6kPa, HCO_3^- 25mmol/L. ★

20. A 60-year-old man is one day post right carotid artery surgery. He suddenly becomes unresponsive with a Glasgow Coma Scale of 8/15. A few minutes later he recovers slightly but is unable to move the left arm or leg. His blood gas results are: pH 7.54, PaO_2 12kPa, $PaCO_2$ 3.6kPa, HCO_3^- 24.3mmol/L. ★★

ANSWERS

Single Best Answers

1. C ★   OH Clin Surg, 4th edn → p52

The management of diabetic patients undergoing major surgery is important. The anaesthetist should be informed and the patient put first on the operating list. For those patients on oral medication, long-acting hypoglycaemics (such as gliclazide) should be omitted preoperatively. Metformin blood sugar levels are monitored regularly and if blood sugar exceeds 15mmol/L then an IV insulin regimen should be started. Moving directly to an insulin regimen is only necessary if the patient is already insulin dependent or is poorly controlled on therapy with unstable blood sugars or where blood sugar can be expected to vary acutely, such as with oral bowel preparation.

2. E ★★   OH Clin Surg, 4th edn → p67

Total parenteral nutrition is commonly encountered on surgical wards for patients in need of nutritional support as a consequence of their underlying disease or following surgery. These patients require regular review and monitoring of their nutritional status by requesting U&E (initially daily then twice weekly once established), glucose (initially daily then twice weekly), LFTs (twice weekly), and micronutrients (Mg, PO_4, Mn, Cu, weekly).

3. B ★★★   OH Clin Surg, 4th edn → p73

Up to 25 000 people per year admitted to hospital in the UK may die from a potentially preventable hospital-acquired venous thromboembolism (VTE). This includes people admitted for both medical conditions and surgery. In order to address this issue the National Institute for Health and Clinical Excellence (NICE) has published guidelines for reducing this risk and it is mandatory for all patients to undergo VTE risk assessment and appropriate treatment. Patients are assessed for their risk of developing VTE and specific interventions are implemented. In this case there is a reduction in mobility due to surgery so thromboprophylaxis is indicated in the form of TED stockings but he has no other risk factors such as malignancy, pelvic surgery, dehydration, older age, or abdominal surgery which would prompt conventional dose low-molecular-weight heparin to be used (5000IU once a day). Thus the patient is low risk and therefore requires TED stockings only.

→ http://www.wales.nhs.uk/sites3/Documents/781/CG92NICE GuidelinePDF.pdf

4. D ★   OH Clin Surg, 4th edn → p73

Prophylactic antibiotics are used to prevent infections in patients undergoing surgery. The type and combination of antibiotics given depend on the type of surgery. For patients undergoing 'clean' bowel surgery, such as acute non-perforated appendicitis, a systemic dose at the time of surgery (ideally given at induction so that the dose is circulating during and immediately after surgery) is usually all that is required. An extended course which should be a full 5 days, is given in circumstances where there is significant contamination or where the risk of sepsis is higher, for example, where an appendix abscess has been found. There are a number of possible alternatives but anaerobic cover should always be part of the treatment for prophylaxis against bowel organisms so metronidazole or similar should be included. Flucloxacillin is ineffective against anaerobic organisms. Most trusts have their own guidelines for antibiotic use and these are usually available on the hospital intranet.

5. C ★★   OH Clin Surg, 4th edn → p84

Stoma is a term applied to an external opening in a lumenated organ. It may be temporary or permanent. There are different types of stomas and each type has certain features that help to identify them. An ileostomy is usually spouted, has prominent mucosal folds, tends to be dark pink or red in colour (as here), and most commonly is sited in the right iliac fossa although the site is the least predictive feature. A jejunostomy is much more commonly found in the upper abdomen and usually produces very liquid green output. A colostomy more usually produces brown semisolid material and is usually not spouted or only very slightly so. A urostomy looks identical to an end ileostomy but produces only clear yellow urine. There is clearly only one lumen so it is most likely to be an end ileostomy.

6. D ★   OH Clin Surg, 4th edn → p98

This patient must be assumed to have had a transfusion reaction. It may be as a result of rapid destruction (haemolysis) of the donor red blood cells by host antibodies, usually related to ABO blood group incompatibility. The most common cause is clerical error (i.e. the wrong unit of blood being given to the patient). Symptoms and signs include fever and chills, back pain, pink or red urine (haemoglobinuria), hypotension, tachycardia, breathlessness, and tachypnoea. The scenario may be an allergic reaction or a very pronounced febrile response but the transfusion must be stopped. Once this is done resuscitation in the form of oxygen and IV fluids can commence and then measures taken to identify the cause, such as sending the blood unit for analysis and blood cultures.

7. E ★★★   OH Clin Surg, 4th edn → p102

The most likely diagnosis in this case is secondary haemorrhage at the site of anastomosis in the groin. This is usually due to a postoperative infection and typically occurs up to 10 days post surgery. In vascular cases where this occurs the first thing to do is to call for senior help as urgent surgical exploration may be indicated and the situation may deteriorate rapidly with rupture of the wound and major haemorrhage being possible. Once senior help has been alerted, compression of the site will reduce the risk of major bleeding and an angiogram may help confirm the diagnosis. Clotting assessment will be necessary prior to any treatment and obviously any anticoagulation is contraindicated until the bleeding has been dealt with.

8. A ★★★   OH Clin Surg, 4th edn → p112

The first thing to do in these situations is to check that the urinary catheter is not the problem. It may be obstructed, bypassing, or malpositioned. Once the catheter is addressed the patient should be assessed clinically to establish whether they are underfilled or overfilled and managed appropriately.

9. B ★★★   OH Clin Surg, 4th edn → p118

The management of postoperative patients on anticoagulants depends on why they are warfarinized and if they have any active bleeding. The patient is at risk of bleeding complications unless the international normalized ratio is corrected quickly so simply omitting warfarin is not enough. In this case the most appropriate treatment is to give 10mg of vitamin K and recommence warfarin once the international normalized ratio is in the normal range. 1mg is an inadequate dose. Fresh frozen plasma is expensive and short lived in effect; it is only used where there is active or surgical bleeding risk.

10. E ★★   OH Clin Surg, 4th edn → p50

The advice usually given to patients on an oestrogen-only oral contraceptive pill is to stop taking it a month prior to elective surgery. Swapping to a progesterone-only pill is unrealistic and a GP consultation is unlikely in this time frame. These situations are sometimes encountered in the pre-admission clinic and the most appropriate course of action is to inform a more senior member of the team. The oestrogen-only oral contraceptive pill does put up her risk of thromboembolic complications slightly and it may depend on how extensive and prolonged the surgery is anticipated to be to whether this additional risk is acceptable or whether the surgery should be deferred.

11. B ★   OH Clin Surg, 4th edn → pp110–11

The most likely diagnosis is aspiration pneumonia. This is usually due to aspiration of gastric content leading initially to chemical pneumonitis which if not recognized and treated appropriately can lead to a secondary bacterial infection. It is most commonly seen in the apical segments of the right lower lobe. The presence of a nasogastric tube may help to reduce the risk of aspiration by keeping the stomach empty but it also reduces the gag reflex by its presence in the hypopharynx and may worsen aspiration of contents if reflux occurs.

Atelectasis is a more generalized phenomenon and is less likely to be so focal unless there is superadded pneumonia and consolidation.

The X-ray does not show the features of widespread interstitial fluid which would characterize pulmonary oedema or the infiltrates of ARDS.

Pulmonary embolism may give this clinical picture but often has no obvious finding on a chest X-ray.

→ http://www.surgical-tutor.org.uk/default-home.htm

12. B ★   OH Clin Surg, 4th edn → p122

The ASA grade is the most commonly used grading system which accurately predicts morbidity and mortality. There are five ASA grades, as shown in Table 1.1.

Table 1.1 ASA Physical Status Classification System

I	Normal healthy individuals
II	Mild systemic disease without limitation of activity
III	Systemic disease with limitation of activity
IV	Systemic disease that poses a threat to life
V	Systemic disease leading to the patient not being expected to survive 24h with or without surgery

In this case the patient has well-controlled asthma on inhalers and thus has an ASA grade of II.

→ http://www.asahq.org/For-Members/Clinical-Information/ASA-Physical-Status-Classification-System.aspx

13. D ★★   OH Clin Surg, 4th edn → p62

Status epilepticus is defined as either a seizure that lasts 30min, or a series of seizures without consciousness being regained in between.

Although all the given options are part of the management of status epilepticus the single most important first step is to establish a clear airway by either removing an obstruction (e.g. dentures) and/or inserting a Guedel or nasopharyngeal airway. Remember your Advanced Life Support (ALS) guidelines ABC.

14. C ★★ OH Clin Surg, 4th edn → p104

Pseudomonas aeruginosa is an aerobic Gram-negative bacillus that inhabits the gastrointestinal (GI) tract. It is an important cause of hospital-acquired infections especially in patients with a serious underlying condition, e.g. burns. Typical evidence of infection due to this organism includes a blue/green exudate and a sweet/fruity odour.

Escherichia coli mostly commonly infects wounds where there has been direct contamination with intestinal contents, e.g. post appendicectomy or post laparotomy.

Proteus is rarely seen outside the urinary tract but can infect open wounds with dead tissue such as severe burns. It produces a characteristic fish-like odour.

Staphylococcus aureus and *Streptococcus pyogenes* both cause skin-related infections, both primary and secondary, but produce a golden and a simple grey-yellow pus respectively.

15. B ★★★ OH Clin Surg, 4th edn → p54

The rhythm strip in Figure 1.3 shows atrial fibrillation. This is a common arrhythmia that occurs in 5–10% of patients over the age of 65. It is caused by a raised atrial pressure, increased atrial muscle mass, atrial fibrosis, or inflammation and infiltration of the atrium. In the context of a surgical patient the key acute causes are: sepsis, low serum potassium, and myocardial ischaemia. In the context of a patient who has an intra-abdominal anastomosis, leakage and sepsis must be high on the list of causes and thus CT scanning and IV antibiotics feature in the management but this patient's status is severely compromised by the atrial fibrillation which must be dealt with. NICE developed guidelines in 2006 for the management of atrial fibrillation as it occurs in emergency, primary, postoperative, and secondary care. For postoperative patients the guidelines state that 'In patients with a life-threatening deterioration in haemodynamic stability following the onset of atrial fibrillation, emergency electrical cardioversion should be performed, irrespective of the duration of the atrial fibrillation'. Thus in this situation cardioversion is the most appropriate management option and oral treatments such as beta blockers and digoxin are not adequate.

→ http://www.nice.org.uk/nicemedia/live/10982/30052/30052.pdf

16. A ★★★ OH Clin Surg, 4th edn → pp60–1

In order to assess the risk of surgery posed to patients with liver disease a number of classification methods have been developed based on Child's grading which takes into account the presence of jaundice, ascites, encephalopathy, and the level of serum albumin. Based on these, patients fall into one of three groups: A (minimal risk), B (moderate risk), and C (advanced risk). See Table 1.2.

Table 1.2 Risk of surgery posed to patients with liver disease

A (minimal risk)	B (moderate risk)	C (advanced risk)
Serum bilirubin <20mg/L	Serum bilirubin 20–30mg/L	Serum bilirubin >30mg/L
Serum albumin >35g/L	Serum albumin 30–35g/L	Serum albumin <30g/L
No ascites	Controlled ascites	Uncontrolled ascites
No focal neurology	Minimal neurological dysfunction	Coma
Excellent nutrition	Good nutrition	Cachexia

17. D ★★★★   OH Clin Surg, 4th edn → p76

The distribution of the numbness is classic for the radial nerve distribution. Nerve injury does occur due to poor patient positioning or application of equipment during surgery and is a major cause of clinical negligence claims. Thus it is always important to ensure that patients are positioned correctly and that bony prominences and areas of thin skin are well padded. Also when using a tourniquet on a limb it is important to apply adequate padding before it is inflated. The radial nerve lies against the periosteum of the humerus in the spiral groove and direct pressure from the edge of the tourniquet is most likely to have caused local damage to the nerve. The median and ulnar nerves are less susceptible due to their position within a muscular compartment.

18. C ★★   OH Clin Surg, 4th edn → p115

Clostridium difficile is a Gram-positive rod which is present as one of the 'normal' bacteria in the gut of up to 3% of healthy adults. Patients who have been treated with broad-spectrum antibiotics are at greatest risk of *C. difficile*-associated disease. In addition, risks of contracting *C. difficile* are raised for patients who are elderly, have a serious underlying illness that compromises their immune system, have a prolonged stay in hospital, or have recently had GI surgery. Between 1999 and 2007 there was a significant increase in the reported number of cases of *C. difficile* prompting the NHS to take certain measures, including changes to antibiotic regimens and promoting hand washing. The green offensive diarrhoea is typical but the diagnosis is confirmed by stool assay for *C. difficile* toxin and treatment is usually with oral metronidazole or vancomycin.

Escherichia coli is a normal commensal but may be pathogenic and occasionally potentially fatally so (e.g. *E. coli* O157). *Salmonella* and *Shigella* are also Gram-negative rods that cause infectious diarrhoea and dysentery in severe cases but this is more likely to be brown and watery or even blood-stained rather than green. *Campylobacter* produces profuse watery diarrhoea. All are caught by the faecal–oral transmission route and are not precipitated by antibiotic treatment.

19. B ★★★★   OH Clin Surg, 4th edn → p122

CPAP machines were initially used mainly by patients for the treatment of sleep apnoea at home, but now are in widespread use across intensive care units as a form of ventilation. CPAP provides a continuous standing airway pressure throughout all phases of respiration. It can be applied via a face mask to a spontaneously breathing patient. It can be used in exhausted patients with chronic obstructive pulmonary disease as is the case with this patient. This patient already has supplemental oxygenation and further increases are unlikely to deal with the deterioration in his status. Any form of positive pressure ventilation may increase oxygenation to some degree but the barotrauma to the lung parenchyma and airways can worsen the situation and make the chances of 'weaning' off ventilation poor.

20. E ★★★   OH Clin Surg, 4th edn → p110

There are a number of causes that may lead to hyperkalaemia (K^+ >5.0–5.5mmol/L) in surgical patients. Renal failure (pre-renal, renal, post-renal), tissue necrosis, and medication (potassium-sparing diuretics) are the leading causes. If the potassium is >6mmol/L then this needs to be treated. An ECG is an important part of patient management and may show signs such as flattened P waves, wide QRS complex, and tented T waves. It is important to repeat the U&E before instigating treatment which includes giving calcium gluconate, actrapid, and calcium resonium.

21. D ★★   OH Clin Surg, 4th edn → p220

Local anaesthetic toxicity is caused by an overdose of local anaesthetic, with systemic absorption, or by accidental IV injection. The systemic toxic effects primarily involve the central nervous system and cardiovascular system. In general the central nervous system is more sensitive to local anaesthetic than the cardiovascular system thus central nervous system manifestations tend to occur earlier.

Early or mild toxicity: light-headedness, dizziness, tinnitus, circumoral numbness, abnormal taste, confusion, and drowsiness. Patients often will not volunteer information about these symptoms unless asked. Throughout the injection talk to the patient, asking them how they feel. Any suggestion of confusion should alert you to the possibility of toxicity and you should stop any further injection.

Severe toxicity: tonic–clonic convulsion leading to progressive loss of consciousness, coma, respiratory depression, and respiratory arrest.

Treatment is based on the ABCD of Basic Life Support.

→ http://www.aagbi.org/sites/default/files/la_toxicity_2010.pdf

22. **E** ★   OH Clin Surg, 4th edn → p201

Surgical emphysema is a condition where air is present in the subcutaneous tissue. It has a characteristic crackling feel to the touch, a sensation that has been described as similar to touching Rice Krispies or tissue paper. Its most common causes are following laparoscopic surgery where CO_2 escapes into the tissues around port sites (e.g. abdominal wall) but pathological causes include pneumothorax and an improperly functioning chest drain. Chest drains have a tendency to form a clot in them or become occluded with fibrinous material. In the setting of an air leak, when chest tube occlusion or clogging occurs, surgical emphysema will occur.

A haemothorax is unlikely since it would usually have occurred as a result of the trauma or on insertion of the chest drain and thus be present from insertion. There is no reason for a pleural effusion or empyema to have formed and neither will give rise to crepitus.

Pulmonary oedema may form areas of trauma although these are localized and usually mixed with blood (pulmonary contusion).

23. **D** ★   OH Clin Surg, 4th edn → pp208–9

When inserting a fine-bore feeding tube the location of the tube must be confirmed before any feeding is started. Aspirating stomach content and blowing air down the tube that can be heard on auscultation of the stomach are often used when large-bore nasogastric tubes are inserted but are both ultimately unreliable and a low pH and air sounds may be heard even if the tube is not within the stomach. Nothing should be put down the tube, even saline since this could be passing directly into the bronchial tree. A chest X-ray must be done to exclude inadvertent bronchial intubation before commencement of feeding, especially in fine-bore tubes.

24. **C** ★   OH Clin Surg, 4th edn → p70

Anxiolytic premedication is still widely used by anaesthetists to reduce anxiety and stress prior to general anaesthesia since it may reduce both intraoperative and postoperative anaesthetic and analgesic requirements. Premedication is no longer used to reduce respiratory secretions (e.g. buscopan) or to reduce reaction to anaesthetic agents (e.g. chlorpheniramine). Opiates have significant side effects and a benzodiazepine is the most likely drug of choice. Midazolam is short acting and will largely have worn off by the time of theatre.

Extended Matching Questions

1. F ★★★ OH Clin Surg, 4th edn → p40

Assessment of aortic calibre can be performed by ultrasound scan or CT scanning but for population screening the lack of radiation exposure means that ultrasound scanning is the method of choice. Simple transabdominal scanning is required and colour flow duplex assessment is not necessary since it is only aortic size that is measured.

2. I ★ OH Clin Surg, 4th edn → p38

Pelvic pathology, especially pathologies related to cystic change of fluid, is best investigated with ultrasound. CT scanning would likely detect an ovarian cyst but there is associated radiation exposure which is best avoided in a woman of this age. Transvaginal scanning is superior to transabdominal scanning especially for subtle pelvic disease.

3. D ★★★ OH Clin Surg, 4th edn → p38

The most likely pathology causing these symptoms is damage to the anal sphincteric mechanism. Although this can be functionally assessed by anorectal physiology, structural evaluation of the sphincter requires an imaging method. MRI scanning will image the pelvic floor but lacks detailed resolution of the sphincteric structures. Ultrasound scanning is the most useful and it requires endoanal scanning which uses a hard-tipped probe rather than transrectal scanning which uses a water-filled balloon.

4. F ★★ OH Clin Surg, 4th edn → p36

The main differential diagnosis is gallstones. The history is most suggestive of biliary colic and there is no suggestion of stones in the distal common bile duct which can be identified by dedicated biliary MRI scanning (magnetic resonance cholangiopancreatography, MRCP) or endoluminal ultrasound scan. Transabdominal ultrasound is safe and avoids a radiation exposure but if it were to prove negative for gallstones or another clear cause, CT scanning would likely be the second-line investigation.

5. C ★

Venous reflux can be detected using Doppler ultrasound which will detect the change in signal frequency caused by the reversal of flow direction of the venous blood. This is usually converted into a simple audible signal with a hand-held device. Colour flow information (duplex scanning) gives additional information about blood flow velocity and morphology but is not required in this instance.

6. C ★★

Atelectasis most commonly occurs in the first 48h following surgery, especially in patients who undergo upper abdominal surgery and patients who smoke. Treatment includes intensive chest physiotherapy, nebulizers, and antibiotics if there is associated infection.

7. E ★★

Fat embolism may occur whenever there is the opportunity for fat to enter the circulatory system. The commonest causes are trauma where long bones containing marrow are fractured and extensive surgery, especially spinal. Fat emboli may be produced mechanically as large fat droplets are released into the venous system, especially cortical veins in large marrow spaces. These droplets are deposited in the pulmonary capillary beds and travel through arteriovenous shunts to the brain. Alternatively, hormonal changes caused by trauma and/or sepsis may induce systemic release of free fatty acids as chylomicrons which form emboli.

The syndrome presents with pyrexia, tachycardia, tachypnoea, reduced consciousness, and in some cases a petechial rash.

8. A ★★   OH Clin Surg, 4th edn → p98

This is transfusion-related acute lung injury. It is a severe acute reaction characterized by respiratory distress, hypoxia, and pulmonary infiltrates soon after transfusion with no other apparent cause. The incidence of transfusion-related acute lung injury varies from 0.001% to 0.16% per patient transfused.

9. H ★   OH Clin Surg, 4th edn → p121

Pulmonary embolism accounts for 3% of hospital inpatient deaths and if untreated has a mortality of 30% compared to 2% when treated appropriately. Patients may present with dyspnoea, pleuritic chest pain, and haemoptysis. Only about 10% will have clinical evidence of a deep venous thrombosis.

10. G ★

One recognized complication of central line insertion is a pneumothorax. A chest X-ray should be requested following the procedure to check the position of the line and to exclude a pneumothorax.

11. E ★   OH Clin Surg, 4th edn → p78

High concentrations of alcohol are extremely effective disinfectants provided the surface treated is allowed to desiccate fully. Most of the other solutions are too caustic for skin surface use. Povidone-iodine solution is rarely used for simple peripheral line insertion but can be used during central line skin preparation. Cationic soap solution will foam up and will prevent the dressing from adhering to the skin

12. A ★★★   OH Clin Surg, 4th edn → p78

Acetaldehyde solution is ideal for cleaning surgical instruments which have inaccessible areas which require disinfection (e.g. the working channels of the scope) since it has very low viscosity and is easily rinsed clear with water (unlike povidone-iodine, aqueous alcohol gel, organic dyes or soap solutions) and which are too delicate to undergo heat treatment (e.g. autoclaving), irradiation, or be subject to caustic substances such as chloroxylenol or peroxide.

13. C ★★   OH Clin Surg, 4th edn → p78

Skin disinfection is best performed with a soap-based product since cleansing the skin surface of dirt and loose skin is assisted by the action of soap. Alcoholic povidone-iodine lacks soap and repeated use of chloroxylenol may cause a skin reaction and is not used for skin cleansing. The others are too caustic for skin surface use.

14. G ★★   OH Clin Surg, 4th edn → p78

In this circumstance the optimum disinfectant would be able to penetrate the small channels of the lateral tracks thus not only should it have a very low viscosity (which precludes organic dye preparations, povidone-iodine, soap solutions, and aqueous alcohol gel), it must be safe to use on exposed body tissue (which excludes chloroxylenol). The effervescence of hydrogen peroxide solution on contact with proteins which causes oxidation producing oxygen, helps to drive it into small tracks and crevices.

15. I ★★★   OH Clin Surg, 4th edn → p78

The ideal combination for a skin preparation agent is a chemically active agent in alcohol solution. Alcohol alone can be used but not at 100% concentration. Simple aqueous solutions are less effective than alcoholic. The commonest skin preps for surgery are povidone-iodine and chlorhexidine in alcoholic solution (but not in aqueous soap form).

16. A ★★

17. G ★★

18. D ★★

19. I ★

20. H ★★

General feedback on 16–20: OH Clin Surg, 4th edn → p94

The body is continually producing acid as a by-product of metabolism. However, it must also maintain a narrow range of pH values necessary for normal enzymic activity. This narrow range of pH values is maintained by intracellular and extracellular buffers and then by the kidneys and lungs. The most important buffer system in the body is the carbonic acid–bicarbonate system: $H_2O + CO_2 \leftrightarrow H_2CO_3 \leftrightarrow HCO_3^- + H^+$

Unlike other buffer systems, the components of the carbonic acid–bicarbonate system can be varied independently of each other. Adjusting the rate of alveolar ventilation changes carbon dioxide (CO_2) concentrations, and the kidneys regulate secretion of protons (H^+) in urine. The excretory functions of the lungs and kidneys are connected by H_2CO_3 (carbonic acid). This is the respiratory–metabolic link. If the kidneys or lungs become overwhelmed, the other can help or 'compensate'. There are four possible primary acid–base disorders—respiratory acidosis, caused by ineffective ventilation; respiratory alkalosis, caused by over-ventilation; metabolic acidosis, caused by an overwhelming acid load or kidney problems; and metabolic alkalosis, caused by an overwhelming base load or dehydration. Table 1.3 gives a summary.

Table 1.3 Changes in pH, $PaCO_2$, and standard bicarbonate in the different acid–base disturbances

	Uncompensated			Compensated		
	pH	$PaCO_2$	Standard bicarbonate	pH	$PaCO_2$	Standard bicarbonate
Respiratory acidosis	Low	High	Normal–high	Normal–low	High	High
Respiratory alkalosis	High	Low	Normal	Normal–high	Low	Low
Metabolic acidosis	Low	Normal	Low	Normal–low	Low	Low
Metabolic alkalosis	High	Normal	High	Normal–high	High	High

Chapter 2

Surgical pathology

Serena Ledwidge

Understanding of the fundamental processes of pathology is essential both to the understanding of how many surgical conditions arise and develop and to the vital role of appreciating the principles of how best to treat conditions. For example, the nature and behaviour of infecting organisms determines whether radical debridement of tissue or simple surgical drainage is required; the stage and grade of tumours influence not only the choice of surgical procedure but the use of adjuvant therapies. These 'surgical' pathologies are often seen as rather 'old-fashioned' compared to the emphasis on cell and molecular biology so often found in books describing medical specialities but they form the bulk of the processes of disease suffered worldwide and remain fundamental to the skilled practice of surgery today.

Neil Borley

QUESTIONS

Single Best Answers

1. A 42-year-old gardener has an infected calf wound caused by an injury with a garden fork. Which *single* feature would indicate that his wound is healing by secondary intention? ★

A Capillary proliferation

B Fibrin precipitation to bridge wound edges

C Fibroblast secretion of elastin

D Formation of granulation tissue

E Thrombosis in cleanly cut blood vessels

2. A 9-year-old boy falls from a swing in the playground and suffers a laceration to his knee. Which *single* sequela of acute inflammation results in formation of granulation tissue? ★

A Degeneration

B Fibrosis

C Organization

D Resolution

E Suppuration

3. A 33-year-old man has had intermittent bloody diarrhoea, weight loss, and colicky abdominal pains for 6 years. A barium meal and follow through shows transmural oedema of the small bowel wall, mucosal ulceration, and skip lesions. Steroids are prescribed. Which *single* pathological feature is pathognomonic of the disease suggested by this history? ★★

A Decreased vascular permeability

B Granuloma formation

C Mesenteric haemorrhage

D Mucosal fibrinous exudate

E Pseudomembranous colitis

4. A 35-year-old woman has dyspnoea, a patchy erythematous rash on her legs, enlarged lymph nodes, and hilar lymphadenopathy on chest X-ray. A lymph node biopsy confirms a granulomatous disease. With which *single* type of cell is a granuloma most likely to be associated? ★★

A Fibroblast

B Histiocyte

C Lymphocyte

D Monocyte

E Neutrophil

5. A 65-year-old woman with chronic leg ulcers and cellulitis for which she has been taking antibiotics for 4 weeks is admitted to hospital for inpatient care. She develops diarrhoea. Her diarrhoea is most likely to be associated with which *single* macroscopic appearance of acute inflammation of the intestine? ★

A Catarrhal

B Fibrinous

C Haemorrhagic

D Pseudomembranous

E Suppurative

6. A 26-year-old glazier sustains a clean laceration to his right forearm. One week after his injury, fibroblasts migrate into the wound to synthesize collagen. Which *single* term best describes his current stage of wound healing? ★

A Fibrosis

B Haemostasis

C Inflammation

D Maturation

E Proliferation

7. A 62-year-old man with type 1 diabetes develops rapidly spreading inflammation with cellulitis and tissue loss of the lower abdominal wall and scrotum as a result of synergistic bacterial infection. Which *single* macroscopic appearance of inflammation is most likely to describe this condition? ★

A Fibrinous

B Haemorrhagic

C Membranous

D Necrotizing

E Suppurative

8. A 65-year-old woman with osteoarthritis of the hip is admitted to hospital for a total hip replacement. Her regular medications include aspirin, alfacalcidol, and prednisolone. Which *single* factor is most likely to result in impaired wound healing? ★

A Corticosteroid

B Non-steroidal anti-inflammatory drugs (NSAIDs)

C Vitamin C deficiency

D Vitamin D deficiency

E Zinc deficiency

9. A 22-year-old medical student suffers a needlestick injury after taking a blood sample from a patient who is an intravenous drug user. She asks about her risk of contracting blood-borne viruses. Which is the *single* most appropriate advice? ★★★

A Chronic infection with hepatitis C is prevalent in 1% of the UK population

B Enzyme-linked immunosorbent assay (ELISA) tests for HIV antibodies are reliably effective 1 month following exposure

C Post-exposure prophylaxis reduces the risk of HIV seroconversion by over 80% if started within 1h of exposure

D Risk of contracting HIV from a hollow needlestick injury is 3%

E Transmission of hepatitis B from a contaminated sharps injury occurs in 10% of cases

10. A 60-year-old woman asks for advice about bowel cancer screening. Her elder brother has recently been diagnosed with bowel cancer and she would like to know about screening tests. She currently has no symptoms, and there is no other family history. Which is the *single* most appropriate advice? ★★★

A A positive faecal occult blood test would mean a >50% chance of having an underlying colorectal cancer

B Colonoscopy is offered to all patients screened

C She is ineligible as screening is offered to males only

D She is ineligible as screening is offered to patients over 65

E Screening is repeated every 2 years for eligible patients

11. A 48-year-old woman has a non-tender but disfiguring soft, round swelling overlying her left scapula. She would like it removed. A junior medical student asks which characteristic or examination technique can best differentiate between a cystic lesion and a lipoma. Which is the *single* most appropriate advice? ★

A Aspiration

B Fluctuation

C Palpation

D Percussion

E Transillumination

12. A 78-year-old woman who developed an extensive deep vein thrombosis in her 50s has a 15cm venous ulcer in the gaiter area of her leg, just above the lateral malleolus which has been present for 10 years. During the last 4 months new tissue which is friable and bleeds has formed within the ulcer. Which *single* feature on examination of the ulcer is most likely to suggest malignant change? ★★

A Base: bleeding granulation tissue

B Edge: everted

C Local lymph nodes: firm and enlarged

D Site: gaiter area

E Size: >10cm

13. A 73-year-old man with a 40-pack-year history has pain in his calf, thigh, and buttock on walking, which is relieved by resting. He suddenly develops a cold, painful white leg. A medical student asks about the acute vascular cause of his symptoms. Which *single* statement is correct? ★★

A An embolus is a solid collection of blood cells within a fibrin network

B Arterial thrombosis requires disruption of blood vessel endothelium, disruption of blood flow, and changes in blood constituents

C Atherosclerosis involves the development of fibrolipid plaques which progress to form fatty streaks and complex lesions

D Phlegmasia alba dolens results from ilio-femoral arterial thrombosis

E Propagation of thrombus involves growth in the direction of blood flow

14. A 65-year-old woman who has had intermittent constipation for years develops a constant lower left abdominal pain and swinging pyrexia. She has rebound tenderness in the left iliac fossa. Her white cell count is 21×10^9/L. Which is the *single* most appropriate statement? ★★★

A A labelled white cell scan is the most appropriate investigation

B Antibiotics are the treatment of choice for diverticular abscess

C Hartmann's procedure results in an end colostomy which is reversible

D Perforation of a diverticulum always results in faecal contamination

E Pneumaturia is a clinical feature of a diverticular abscess

15. A 35-year-old man has noticed a 1cm diameter non-tender lump in his scrotum, separate from the testis but palpable within the epididymis. Which is the *single* most appropriate description of the most likely pathological finding? ★★

A Acquired distension cyst

B Acquired retention cyst

C Congenital sequestration dermoid

D Congenital tubulo-embryonic cyst

E Dilated vestigial remnant

16. A 28-year-old hirsute man has a painful inflamed area in the natal cleft between his buttocks from which there has been recent purulent discharge from follicular pits, as shown in Figure 2.1.

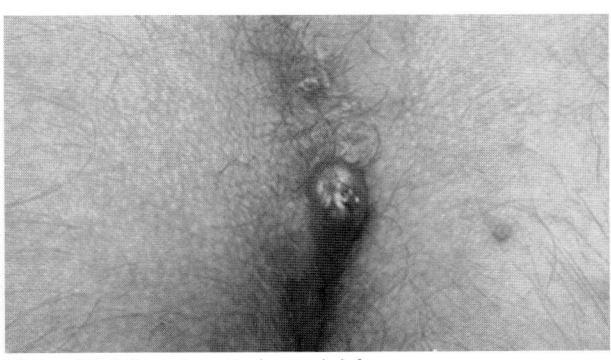

Figure 2.1 Inflamed area in the natal cleft

Which is the *single* most appropriate statement? ★★★

A A sinus is an abnormal communication between two epithelial surfaces

B A sinus tract is lined by granulation tissue

C Sinus formation in this area is associated with ulcerative colitis

D The tract is likely to communicate with the anorectum

E Treatment of the sinus involves the use of a seton

17. A 62-year-old man with heartburn and acid reflux since his 40s develops weight loss and dysphagia to solids. Endoscopy demonstrates a distal oesophageal carcinoma. CT scan shows local tumour invasion and liver metastases. With respect to cellular changes underlying his malignancy, which *single* statement is correct? ★★

A Barrett's oesophagus is a dysplastic change of the epithelial lining of the oesophagus

B Barrett's oesophagus leads to oesophageal squamous cell carcinoma

C Metaplasia represents an adaptive tissue response to an environmental stress

D Metastasis involves the secretion of proteolytic enzymes which weaken normal connective tissue bonds

E The tumour is likely to be encapsulated

18. A 42-year-old construction worker treated in the intensive care unit following a severe crush injury of his lower left leg develops gas gangrene of the limb. Which is the *single* most appropriate statement? ★

A A 'watch and wait' policy should be followed until a zone of demarcation appears between dead and living tissues over a period of days

B Broad-spectrum antibiotics should not be commenced to avoid masking the spread of the gangrene

C Intraoperatively, any tissue that is questionably viable should be left *in situ*, in order to minimize tissue loss

D Pus in the tissues should be aspirated percutaneously

E Urgent amputation and debridement of necrotic tissue is indicated

Extended Matching Questions

Cell/tissue death

For each scenario choose the *single* most appropriate pathological term describing cell or tissue death from the list of options. Each option may be used once, more than once, or not at all.

A Apoptosis

B Caseous necrosis

C Coagulative necrosis

D Colliquative necrosis

E Dry gangrene

F Fat necrosis

G Fibrinoid necrosis

H Necrotizing fasciitis

I Wet gangrene

1. A 35-year-old woman with a firm lump in the breast who bumped into the corner of a wardrobe 1 month previously. ★★

2. A 46-year-old Asian man with a past history of tuberculosis has a matted mass of cervical lymph nodes with a cheesy macroscopic appearance. ★

3. A 67-year-old man, with a dense hemiplegia, who suffered a thrombotic stroke 1 week ago. ★

4. A 67-year-old hypertensive woman with death of vascular smooth muscle cells local to an atherosclerotic plaque causing a 70% internal carotid artery stenosis. ★★

5. A 70-year-old smoker with a 50-pack-year history has rest pain in his foot, a desiccated blackened 4th toe, and an ulcer on the neighbouring toe. ★

6. A 38-year-old man with type 1 diabetes who has a blackened hallux with cellulitis and bogginess in the surrounding tissue. ★

Tumours

For each scenario choose the *single* most likely primary tumour from the list of options. Each option may be used once, more than once, or not at all.

A Astrocytoma

B Basal cell carcinoma

C Colorectal adenocarcinoma

D Hodgkin's lymphoma

E Melanoma

F Non-Hodgkin's lymphoma

G Seminoma

H Squamous cell carcinoma

I Thyroid follicular carcinoma

7. A 67-year-old man with groin lymphadenopathy and a fungating lesion at his anal margin. ★

8. A 73-year-old man with a penetrating ulcer in his inner nasal canthus. ★

9. A 43-year-old woman who had her hallux amputated for a subungual lesion in her 30s develops a retinal metastasis. ★

10. A 35-year-old man has a chest X-ray which shows 'cannonball' lesions. ★

11. A 55-year-old man with a palpable liver edge and raised carcinogenic embryonic antigen. ★

Tumour markers

For each scenario choose the *single* most appropriate tumour marker from the list of options. Each option may be used once, more than once, or not at all.

A Alpha-fetoprotein (AFP)

B Alkaline phosphatase

C Beta human chorionic gonadotrophin (β-HCG)

D Calcitonin

E CA19-9

F Carcinogenic embryonic antigen

G Lactate dehydrogenase (LDH)

H Placental alkaline phosphatase

I Prostate-specific antigen

12. A 45-year-old Chinese immigrant worker who is a carrier of HBsAg with right upper quadrant pain and a palpable mass. ★★

13. An asymptomatic 36-year-old man who underwent orchidectomy for a testicular seminoma 1 year ago. ★★

14. A 62-year-old woman with weight loss in whom a Whipple's procedure is planned. ★★

15. An 80-year-old man diagnosed with a cancer that is being managed by 'watchful waiting'. ★★

16. A 48-year-old woman with a painless lump in her neck and a hoarse voice who has a recent onset of frequent diarrhoea. ★★

17. A 56-year-old man who has had neoadjuvant therapy prior to anterior resection for a rectal carcinoma. ★★

ANSWERS

Single Best Answers

1. D ★   OH Clin Surg, 4th edn → p147

Wound healing by primary intention takes place where there is close apposition of clean wound edges. Healing by secondary intention occurs when wound edges cannot be cleanly apposed. Capillary proliferation occurs in healing by both primary and secondary intention. Although fibrin is precipitated in healing by secondary intention, this will not bridge the gap between wound edges, and granulation tissue will fill in the tissue defect. Fibroblast secretion of collagen into the fibrin network is involved in primary healing. Thrombosis occurs in disrupted blood vessels, but these are rarely cleanly cut in wound healing by secondary intention.

2. C ★   OH Clin Surg, 4th edn → p145

There are four possible outcomes following acute inflammation: resolution is the restoration of the tissue to normal, suppuration refers to the formation of pus, organization whereby the tissue is repaired, or chronic inflammation. Degeneration is not part of the process of acute inflammation. Fibrosis refers to the formation of fibrous tissue to form a scar.

3. B ★★   OH Clin Surg, 4th edn → p145

The clinical picture is that of Crohn's disease, an inflammatory bowel disease which may affect any part of the alimentary tract and involves the full thickness of the bowel wall in affected segments. Crohn's disease is characterized by the microscopic appearance of granulomas which consist of epithelioid cells and Langhans giant cells. A fibrinous exudate may occur, but characteristically this affects the bowel serosa and may result in matted loops of bowel, predisposing to fistula formation. Mesenteric haemorrhage is not characteristic of this condition, and pseudomembranous colitis, superficial mucosal ulceration of the colon, tends to occur as a response to treatment with antibiotics resulting in secondary infection, e.g. by *Clostridium difficile*.

4. B ★★   OH Clin Surg, 4th edn → p145

A granuloma is an aggregate of epithelioid histiocytes, activated macrophages resembling epithelial cells. The underlying diagnosis is sarcoidosis, characterized by the presence of non-caseating granulomas in affected organ tissues. Neutrophils, monocytes, and lymphocytes are types of leucocyte, fibroblasts are connective tissue cells which make and secrete collagen.

5. D ★ OH Clin Surg, 4th edn → p144

Pseudomembranous colitis may occur after major abdominal surgery but is most often seen as a consequence of antibiotic administration. The causative organism is *Clostridium difficile* and its toxin can be isolated from the stool of over 90% of patients. The mucosal surface of the large bowel has superficial ulceration. Catarrhal inflammation results in mucus hypersecretion, e.g. the common cold. Fibrinous inflammation results in exudates containing fibrin which forms a coating, e.g. pericarditis. Haemorrhagic inflammation results in vascular injury and bleeding, e.g. pancreatitis. Suppurative inflammation involves the formation of pus.

6. E ★ OH Clin Surg, 4th edn → p146

The four stages of wound healing are haemostasis, which occurs immediately due to the presence of exposed collagen resulting in platelet aggregation and degranulation. Thrombus formation is initiated by the clotting and complement cascades. Inflammation occurs between 0 and 3 days after the injury. Proliferation, in which fibroblasts migrate into the wound and secrete collagen, occurs between 3 days and 3 weeks. Angiogenesis is stimulated and granulation tissue forms. Re-orientation and maturation of collagen tissue fibres occurs as part of the remodelling process which occurs between 3 weeks and 1 year.

7. D ★ OH Clin Surg, 4th edn → pp144, 175

This is necrotizing fasciitis or synergistic spreading gangrene, which has the eponyms Meleney's or Fournier's gangrene. The organisms involved are aerobes and microaerophilic/anaerobes. The initial wound may be minor but results in rapidly spreading tissue necrosis. Patients may be immunocompromised. The patient requires systemic resuscitation, antibiotics, and urgent debridement of involved tissues. Membranous inflammation has a coating of fibrin and epithelial cells, e.g. laryngitis. Fibrinous, haemorrhagic, and suppurative inflammation are described in the answer to SBA 5.

8. A ★ OH Clin Surg, 4th edn → p147

Vitamins C and D and zinc are important factors associated with wound healing. NSAIDs suppress inflammation, but long-term steroids have the most significant effect in terms of impaired wound healing.

→ Stadelmann WK, Digenis AG, Tobin GR. Impediments to wound healing. *Am J Surg* 1998; 176(2A Suppl.):39S–47S.

9. C ★★★ OH Clin Surg, 4th edn → p178

The prevalence of HIV in UK injecting drug users is around 1%. ELISA tests for HIV antibodies are only effective and reliable after seroconversion following a 3-month 'window' after infection. The risk of contracting HIV from hollow needlestick injury is 0.3%. Post-exposure prophylaxis with anti-retroviral medication reduces the risk of seroconversion by over 80% if started within 1h of exposure, and should be continued for 4 weeks. The risk of transmission of hepatitis B following contaminated needlestick injury is 30%. Chronic infection with hepatitis C is prevalent in 0.4% of the UK population.

10. E ★★★ OH Clin Surg, 4th edn → pp165–6

The NHS Bowel Cancer Screening Programme offers faecal occult blood testing to men and women aged 60–69 (this may be extended to age 74 in future), and repeated every 2 years. Those testing positive will be offered a colonoscopy. Around one in ten patients who go on to have a colonoscopy will be found to have a cancer.

→ Department of Health. *Bowel Cancer—The Facts*. http://www.cancerscreening.nhs.uk

11. A ★ OH Clin Surg, 4th edn → p150

Aspiration of a cyst will produce fluid. Cysts and lipomas have similar consistency. Both may be fluctuant and transilluminate. Percussion is of little value, but will be dull in both pathologies. In clinical practice, ultrasound is frequently used to differentiate between cysts and lipomas.

12. B ★★ OH Clin Surg, 4th edn → p148

The everted edge is suggestive of the development of a squamous cell carcinoma (Marjolin's ulcer). This may occur in long-term ulceration. Bleeding granulation tissue in the base of an ulcer suggests chronicity and attempts at healing in the presence of an adequate arterial supply: this is not necessarily suggestive of malignancy. Local nodes may well be firm and enlarged as a consequence of reactive lymphadenopathy due to secondary infection of the ulcer. The gaiter area and ulcer size bear no specific risks for malignant change. The edge of a venous ulcer is characteristically flat or sloping.

13. E ★★ OH Clin Surg, 4th edn → pp154–5

An embolus is a mobile mass of material in the vascular system capable of blocking a vessel lumen. This may not necessarily be related to blood components, e.g. fat embolus. Arterial and venous thrombosis occurs in the presence of factors described in Virchow's triad: damage to vessel wall, disruption of blood flow, changes in blood constituents. However, not all these changes are required to be present simultaneously for thrombosis to occur. In atherosclerosis, fatty streaks precede the formation of fibrolipid plaques. Phlegmasia alba dolens is a chronic condition referring to painful white leg caused by slow formation of ilio-femoral venous thrombosis.

14. C ★★★   OH Clin Surg, 4th edn → p176

The findings in this patient suggest the presence of a diverticular abscess. The most appropriate investigation to confirm this diagnosis would be a CT scan. Antibiotics are used for first-line treatment of diverticulitis but abscesses require radiological or surgical drainage. Hartmann's procedure involves resection of the sigmoid colon with formation of an end colostomy. This is potentially reversible with re-anastomosis, usually after several months of recovery from the primary procedure, though this is not appropriate for every patient. Perforated diverticular disease may cause variable contamination within the abdomen (originally classified by Hinchey et al. (1978) though this has undergone subsequent modification). Pneumaturia implies the presence of a colo-vesical fistula.

→ Hinchey EJ, Schaal PG, Richards GK. Treatment of perforated diverticular disease of the colon. *Adv Surg* 1978; 12:85–109.

→ Klarenbeek BR, de Korte N, van der Peet DL, Cuesta MA. Review of current classifications for diverticular disease and a translation into clinical practice. *Int J Colorectal Dis* 2012; 27(2):207–14.

15. B ★★   OH Clin Surg, 4th edn → p150

This patient is likely to have an epididymal cyst. This is an example of a retention cyst and may be caused by cystic degeneration of the paradidymis or the appendix of the epididymis. If uncomfortable, these can be excised. Distension cysts arise as a consequence of exudation or secretion in a closed cavity, e.g. hydrocoele. Tubulo-embryonic cysts are due to abnormal budding of tubular structures, e.g. thyroglossal cysts. Examples of vestigial remnants include the vitello-intestinal duct (Meckel's diverticulum) and hydatid of Morgagni.

16. B ★★★   OH Clin Surg, 4th edn → p151

The diagnosis is a pilonidal sinus; if infected, a pilonidal abscess may form. A sinus is a blind-ended tract lined by granulation tissue. A fistula is an abnormal communication between two epithelial surfaces. Perianal fistula formation may occur in Crohn's but is not associated with ulcerative colitis. A seton is a suture placed in a fistula tract which is progressively tightened to lay open the tract and to encourage granulation and healing. A perianal abscess (but not a pilonidal abscess) may be associated with an underlying fistula, communicating with the anorectum.

17. C ★★   OH Clin Surg, 4th edn → p160

Metaplasia is the reversible transformation of one type of differentiated cell into another: it is an adaptive response to stress. Barrett's oesophagus is metaplastic change from stratified squamous epithelium to columnar epithelium and is associated with an increased risk of oesophageal adenocarcinoma. Encapsulation is a feature of benign neoplasms.

Secretion of proteolytic enzymes facilitates local invasion of tumours through tissue planes, not metastasis which is the process by which primary tumours form secondary tumours at distant sites. Dysplasia is a potentially premalignant condition characterized by increased cell growth, atypical morphology, and altered differentiation. Neoplasia is autonomous growth of abnormal cells after the initiating stimulus has been removed.

18. E ★   OH Clin Surg, 4th edn → p158

Gas gangrene occurs when gangrene is infected by gas-producing anaerobic organisms such as *Clostridium perfringens*. Spread of gangrene is usually rapid and requires urgent surgical debridement and broad-spectrum antibiotics, often with 'second-look' surgery. If there is doubt over the viability of the tissue it should be debrided to ensure the gangrene does not spread. Crepitus is associated with surgical emphysema due to necrosis caused by the gas-producing organisms.

Extended Matching Questions

1. F ★★   OH Clin Surg, 4th edn → p142

Fat necrosis may occur in response to trauma. Release of extracellular fat causes an inflammatory response, fibrosis, and, occasionally, a palpable mass.

2. B ★   OH Clin Surg, 4th edn → p142

Caseous necrosis lacks structure and is characterized by a macroscopic white cheesy appearance.

3. D ★   OH Clin Surg, 4th edn → p142

Colliquative necrosis occurs in brain tissue due to lack of architecture of surrounding stromal tissue.

4. A ★★   OH Clin Surg, 4th edn → p143

This is pathological apoptosis, resulting in cell-mediated controlled elimination of smooth muscle cells local to the atherosclerotic plaque.

5. E ★   OH Clin Surg, 4th edn → p142

Necrosis with desiccation. If left to mummify the toe may eventually separate spontaneously.

6. I ★   OH Clin Surg, 4th edn → p142

Gangrene with putrefaction due to secondary infection.

7. H ★   OH Clin Surg, 4th edn → pp168–70

This is a classical presentation of an anal squamous cell carcinoma which undergoes lymphatic metastasis to local groin lymph nodes.

8. B ★   OH Clin Surg, 4th edn → pp168–70

Basal cell carcinomas tend to erode into local tissues by direct invasion, but distant metastasis is rare.

9. E ★   OH Clin Surg, 4th edn → pp168–70

Melanomas spread by local metastasis (satellite lesions), by lymphatic spread and by haematogenous spread to distant sites including lung, brain, and retina. Treatment of a subungual melanoma involves digital amputation and may require block dissection of local lymph nodes.

10. G ★   OH Clin Surg, 4th edn → pp168–70

Seminomas spread by lymphatics to the para-aortic and iliac lymph nodes. Late haematogenous spread to liver, lungs, and bone may occur, with a characteristic appearance of lung metastases.

11. C ★   OH Clin Surg, 4th edn → pp168–70

Colorectal cancer may spread locally by direct invasion, to local lymph nodes and by haematogenous spread most commonly to the liver, but also occasionally, for instance, to lungs and bone.

12. A ★★   OH Clin Surg, 4th edn → p171

13. C ★★   OH Clin Surg, 4th edn → p171

14. E ★★   OH Clin Surg, 4th edn → p171

15. I ★★   OH Clin Surg, 4th edn → p171

16. D ★★   OH Clin Surg, 4th edn → p171

17. H ★★   OH Clin Surg, 4th edn → p171

General feedback on 12–17: Tumour markers are proteins or complex molecules produced by normal cells in small amounts but in increased amounts by tumour cells due to changes in cellular function. Some tumours may produce more than one marker: e.g. testicular teratomas may produce AFP and β-HCG; colorectal tumours may produce carcinogenic embryonic antigen and CA19-9, the former being useful in monitoring response to treatment (17). Other uses of tumour markers include screening for disease and detecting recurrence. In (12) the patient is likely to have developed a primary hepatocellular carcinoma for which AFP is a marker. In (13), seminomas may produce β-HCG (in 10% of cases) but rarely produce AFP which may be elevated in association with teratomas and yolk-sac tumours of the testis. CA19-9 is elevated in 80% of cases of patients with pancreatic cancer. Whipple's procedure may be employed in cases of potentially curative resection of a pancreatic carcinoma. Assessment of a prostatic carcinoma may involve measurement of prostate-specific antigen (15): a policy of 'watchful waiting' may be adopted in elderly men in whom it is deemed unlikely that the cancer will advance rapidly. In (16), the patient has symptoms suggestive of a medullary carcinoma of the thyroid which produces calcitonin.

Chapter 3

Practical procedures

Asmaa Al-Alaak

Surgery is, by its very nature, a highly practical discipline and the range of surgical procedures is wider and more complex than ever with the relentless expansion in surgical technologies. There are, however, numerous more minor procedures which are carried out on both surgical and non-surgical patients with which all junior doctors should be familiar. Any of us may be called upon to drain a serious pleural effusion or insert an intravenous or intra-arterial access. The safe performance of such practical procedures is a vital skill for all doctors. This chapter will review and test all aspects of the more commonplace 'surgical' procedures. It is important that all aspects of the procedures are understood from indications, to safe preparation, and the recognition and management of potential complications.

Although learning these procedures may seem rather like learning a list of facts such as complications, remember to go back to the likely effects of each procedure on the physiology of the organ under consideration. This, coupled with knowledge of the key anatomical structures involved, will usually give enough information to pass even close questioning about them!

Neil Borley

QUESTIONS

Single Best Answers

1. A 70-year-old man is in hospital with acute pancreatitis. He has a past history of intermittent palpitations. An admission ECG shows normal sinus rhythm. Two days later he has palpitations, shortness of breath and chest pain. His pulse is 160bpm, blood pressure is 85/60mmHg, and there are bilateral basal crepitations. A repeat ECG shows a supraventricular tachycardia. Which is the *single* most appropriate management? ★★★

A Amiodarone infusion

B Carotid sinus massage

C Catheter ablation

D DC cardioversion

E Verapamil® orally

2. A 47-year-old woman attends pre-admission clinic prior to elective gynaecological surgery. As part of the pre-admission process, routine blood tests are required. A junior medical student asks about the usual anatomy of the venous drainage in the upper limb. Which is the *single* most appropriate description of the commonest arrangement? ★★

A Cephalic vein commences from the medial end of the dorsal venous network

B Cephalic vein drains into the venae comitantes of the brachial artery

C Basilic vein commences from the lateral end of the palmar venous network

D Basilic vein drains into the axillary vein

E Median cubital vein drains into the basilic and cephalic vein in the cubital fossa

3. A 65-year-old woman is 3 days post total hip replacement. She has a temperature of 39°C. Following advice from the microbiologist she is commenced on IV antibiotics. Twenty-four hours later she remains septic with a temperature of 38°C, a pulse rate of 120bpm, and a C-reactive protein (CRP) of 125g/dL. Her IV cannula has tissued. Following three attempts you fail to cannulate the forearm veins of the patient who is distressed. Which is the *single* most appropriate next step in her management? ★

A Attempt cannulation of dorsal foot veins

B Attempt central venous line insertion

C Change IV antibiotics to oral

D Request a central line insertion by the on-call anaesthetist

E Request a senior colleague to attempt peripheral upper limb cannulation

4. A 22-year-old motorcycle driver is involved in a high-speed road traffic collision. At the scene he has lost a lot of blood and on arrival in the resuscitation room he has a blood pressure of 80/55mmHg and a pulse rate of 140bpm. As a member of the on-call trauma team you are asked by the team leader to gain IV access for this patient. Which is the *single* most appropriate access to use in this situation? ★★

A Blue (22G) in an antecubital fossa vein

B Green (18G) in the dorsum of the hand

C Grey (16G) in an antecubital fossa vein

D Triple lumen central line in the internal jugular vein

E White (17G) in the internal jugular vein

5. A 60-year-old man is scheduled for a low anterior resection for a rectal cancer. He has ischaemic heart disease and due to the possible risk of cardiac complications the anaesthetist is planning to admit the patient to the intensive care unit postoperatively. In the anaesthetic room a radial arterial line is required before the patient is anaesthetized. Which is the *single* most appropriate test that should be performed before inserting the arterial line? ★

A Allen test

B Brodie–Trendelenburg test

C Coombs test

D McMurray test

E Tinel test

6. A 75-year-old man is admitted to the emergency department with abdominal distension and increasing shortness of breath. The patient requires endotracheal intubation. The patient is in the resuscitation room with the anaesthetist and anaesthetic assistant prepared and all equipment and drugs ready to hand. Which is the *single* most appropriate *initial* step of the procedure? ★★★★

A Administer IV suxamethonium

B Extend the neck and ask the anaesthetic assistant for cricoid pressure

C Insert the laryngoscope blade and elevate the jaw

D Administer high-flow oxygen via a non-rebreathing device for 2min

E Suction excess pharyngeal saliva and secretions

7. A 65-year-old man is admitted with acute urinary retention. He requires urethral catheterization and you are selecting the appropriate local anaesthetic preparation for use to assist the procedure. Which is the *single* best preparation to use? ★

A Amethocaine 7.7% ointment

B Lidocaine 2% gel with adrenaline (epinephrine) 1:10 000

C Lignocaine 2% aqueous solution

D Lignocaine 2% gel

E Xylocaine 10mg/mL spray

8. A 70-year-old man is 5 days after a prostatectomy. He has had an indwelling urethral catheter since his surgery. The nurse looking after him calls to say that in the last 2h his urine output has been poor and has been anuric for the last hour. Which is the *single* most appropriate next intervention? ★

A Change the catheter over a guidewire

B Flush the catheter with 10mL saline

C Give 250mL of normal saline 0.9% intravenously

D No intervention is required

E Perform a bladder scan by ultrasound on the ward

9. An 85-year-old woman has been admitted with a fractured neck of femur following a fall. She has ischaemic heart disease with previous coronary bypass surgery. Soon after admission to the orthopaedic ward the patient becomes unresponsive and has no palpable pulse. Cardiopulmonary resuscitation is commenced and the patient is attached to the monitor with this rhythm as shown in Figure 3.1.

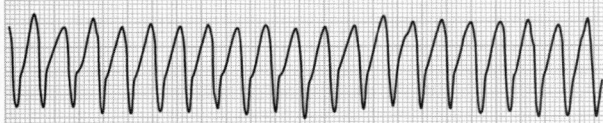

Figure 3.1 The rhythm shown on the monitor during CPR
Reproduced from Longmore et al., *Oxford Handbook of Clinical Medicine*, 8th edition, 2010, with permission from Oxford University Press.

Which is the *single* most appropriate immediate treatment? ★★

A Defibrillate using external defibrillator

B IV adenosine 1mg stat

C IV adrenaline (epinephrine) 10mL of 1:10 000 stat

D IV amiodarone 1g over 4h

E IV lidocaine 100mg over 10min

10. A 37-year-old woman is seen in outpatients and has been passing blood per rectum for 3 months with some anal discomfort and swelling. Verbal consent is taken for a digital rectal examination and rigid sigmoidoscopy in order to complete the clinical assessment. Which is the *single* most accurate description of a likely complication following the procedure? ★

A Anorectal incontinence

B Bradycardia

C Perforation of the caecum

D Rectal bleeding

E Reduced oxygen saturations due to sedation

Extended Matching Questions

Complications of invasive procedures

For each scenario choose the *single* most likely diagnosis from the list of options. Each option may be used once, more than once, or not at all.

A Air embolism

B Arrhythmia

C Arterial puncture

D Arteriovenous fistula

E Brachial plexus injury

F Cardiac tamponade

G Haematoma

H Haemothorax

I Pneumothorax

J Systemic sepsis

K Thoracic duct injury

L Thrombosis of the jugular vein

1. A 50-year-old woman is admitted with a high-output intestinal fistula. She has had a tunnelled central line inserted and has been commenced on total parenteral nutrition. Ten days later she is feeling unwell and feverish. She is flushed and has warm peripheries. Her temperature is swinging up to 38.9°C, heart rate is 120bpm, and blood pressure is 90/50mmHg. ★

2. An 89-year-old woman has been admitted to the intensive care unit with acute renal failure following surgery for a fractured neck of femur. She has a right internal jugular central line inserted as part of her management. She has become rapidly short of breath over a period of 30min with a heart rate rising to 100bpm and blood pressure of 95/80mmHg and cold peripheries. Right-sided breath sounds are reduced and the right chest is dull to percussion. ★

3. A 45-year-old woman has an infected knee replacement. A subclavian line has been inserted for long-term IV antibiotics. Following the procedure she is increasingly short of breath. Her blood pressure is 80/50mmHg, respiratory rate is 26 breaths/min, and heart rate is 117bpm. Her neck veins are dilated and her heart sounds are muffled. An ECG reveals low-voltage QRS complexes. ★★

4. A 75-year-old man has a prolonged ileus following abdominal surgery. He has a central venous line inserted into the right internal jugular vein side for short-term total parenteral nutrition. Following the procedure he has developed numbness down the medial aspect of his forearm and both the little and ring finger. ★

5. A 39-year-old woman is diagnosed with a large breast cancer. She has a central line inserted prior to commencing neoadjuvant chemotherapy. Immediately at the end of the procedure she develops chest pain, a persistent cough, increasing shortness of breath, and she is becoming more confused. Her blood pressure is 70/45mmHg, heart rate is 124bpm and irregular. Inspiration is symmetrical with a normal percussion note and there are widespread fine inspiratory crepitations. Oxygen saturations fall to 88% despite supplemental oxygen. ★★★

Surface anatomical landmarks

For each scenario a practical procedure is required, choose the *single* most appropriate surface anatomical landmark (shown in Figure 3.2) you would use to start the procedure from the list of options. Each option may be used once, more than once, or not at all.

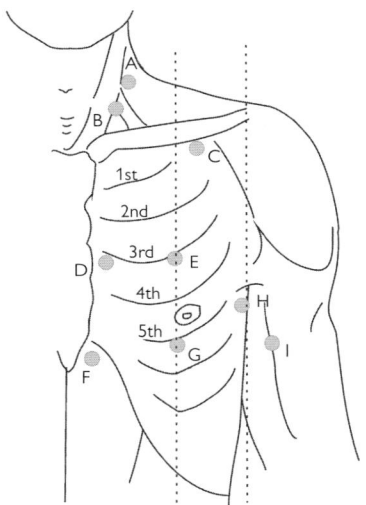

Figure 3.2 Surface anatomical landmarks

A Lateral border of the body of sternocleidomastoid

B Apex of the junction of the clavicular and sternal heads of sternocleidomastoid

C 1cm below the junction of the outer and middle thirds of the clavicle

D Below the left 3rd costal cartilage in the parasternal line

E Below the 3rd rib in the mid-clavicular line

F 1cm below and to the left of the xiphoid process

G 5th intercostal space in the mid-clavicular line

H 5th intercostal space in the mid-axillary line

I Bicipital groove below the tendon of pectoralis major

6. A 58-year-old man with a past history of vascular disease and carotid endarterectomy requires transfer to the intensive care unit with fast atrial fibrillation and requires IV amiodarone treatment and potassium supplementation. Appropriate access is required. ★★

7. A 65-year-old man is having postoperative chemotherapy for a rectal tumour. He requires an indwelling central venous catheter line use over the next 6 months. ★

8. A 24-year-old man sustains a symptomatic pneumothorax following a fall with multiple rib fractures. He requires a chest drain insertion on the ward. ★

9. A 45-year-old man is involved in a severe road traffic collision and has an acute haemopericardium which is compromising his circulation by causing cardiac tamponade. Urgent aspiration/drainage is required. ★★

10. A 72-year-old man has a liver abscess following complicated cholecystitis and microbiological advice is that he should receive 6 weeks of IV antibiotics. Appropriate access is required. ★★

ANSWERS

Single Best Answers

1. D ★★★   OH Clin Surg, 4th edn → p188

Supraventricular tachycardia is usually a narrow complex tachycardia. Manifestations of supraventricular tachycardia are variable; patients may be asymptomatic or may have minor palpitations or more severe symptoms. Control of the rate of a supraventricular tachycardia may be achieved by increasing vagal tone by vagotonic manoeuvres such as carotid sinus massage and chemically with Verapamil® but they are unlikely to result in prompt reversion to sinus rhythm. Patients who are haemodynamically unstable and compromised, as is the case here, should be resuscitated immediately with cardioversion rather than attempting chemical cardioversion with amiodarone which usually takes several hours if not longer.

Catheter ablation is used to destroy re-entry pathways within the cardiac conduction system which cause recurrent, uncontrollable dysrhythmias.

2. E ★★   OH Clin Surg, 4th edn → p193

The cephalic vein commences from the lateral end of the dorsal venous network and the basilic from the medial end. The cephalic vein continues on the lateral aspect of the forearm and arm and drains into the axillary vein deep to the deltoid muscle. The basilic vein drains into the venae comitantes of the brachial artery then drains into the axillary vein. The median cubital vein usually arises out of the cephalic vein and crosses the cubital fossa to drain into the basilic vein.

3. E ★   OH Clin Surg, 4th edn → p195

In these situations it can be stressful for both the doctor and patient. Options to deal with this include taking a short break and trying again a little while later. If you are still unable to cannulate then call a more senior member of your team. A central line is an option but is associated with a higher rate of complications than peripheral access. If required, the line should be performed by somebody trained in ultrasound-guided central venous cannulation and not on the ward without assistance. The dorsal veins of the foot should only be used where even senior help has failed to achieve upper limb cannulation and where central line access is undesirable since they increase the risk of deep vein thrombosis and severely limit patient mobility. Stopping the IV antibiotics in this situation is not appropriate.

4. C ★★   OH Clin Surg, 4th edn → p193

For rapid IV fluid resuscitation in an emergency setting the fastest infusion rate is needed and the flow rate of the cannula is proportional to the radial size (large gauge numbers are the smallest bore) and inversely proportional to length. Thus a triple lumen central line is far too long to be a fast access line. A 17G cannula or larger is required. It doesn't matter where the cannula is sited provided it is not distal to a limb injury which will interfere with flow but the large upper limb veins (such as the antecubital fossa veins) are often easier to access in an emergency.

5. A ★ OH Clin Surg, 4th edn → p197

The hand is normally supplied by blood from the ulnar and radial arteries and they form anastomoses in the hand. Thus, if the blood supply from one of the arteries is cut off, the other artery can supply adequate blood to the hand. In about 3% of patients there is a lack of collateral flow. Thus an Allen test is used to test this collateral blood supply prior to insertion of an arterial line or prior to heart bypass surgery (radial artery is used as a conduit).

Steps involved in the test are:

1. The hand is elevated and the patient/person is asked to make a fist for about 30sec.
2. Pressure is applied over the ulnar and the radial arteries so as to occlude both of them.
3. Still elevated, the hand is then opened. It should appear blanched (pallor can be observed at the finger nails).
4. Ulnar pressure is released and the colour should return in 7sec.

If the colour returns then ulnar artery supply to the hand is sufficient and it is safe to cannulate the radial artery. If colour does not return or returns after 7–10sec, then the ulnar artery supply to the hand is not sufficient and the radial artery therefore cannot be safely cannulated.

A Tinel test is for sensitivity of the median nerve on percussion over the flexor retinaculum.
A Coombs test is a haematological test for agglutination.
A Brodie–Trendelenburg test is for identification of hip abductor weakness during standing on one leg.
A McMurray test is a test for meniscal tenderness after injury.

6. D ★★★★ OH Clin Surg, 4th edn → p186

Endotracheal intubation is indicated in a number of clinical scenarios. The first step is to ensure that the patient is fully pre-oxygenated before commencing the procedure. It does not take long but maximizes the circulating PaO_2 and blood oxygenation which is what the patient is dependent on during the period of loss of respiration needed for the access and insertion procedure prior to re-establishing ventilation.

Depending on the technique used the appropriate muscle relaxant agent (e.g. suxamethonium) is administered but if the intubation is a rapid sequence (emergency) one or if the patient is not starved then cricoid pressure is required before any drugs are administered to reduce the risk of reflux of oesophageal contents. The pharynx can only be suctioned once the patient is anaesthetized and laryngoscopy directly precedes attempted endotracheal intubation.

7. D ★ OH Clin Surg, 4th edn → pp210, 218

Topical local anaesthesia is used for many practical procedures. Lidocaine, lignocaine, and xylocaine are all synonyms for the same compound but the terms are all still widely used in drug preparations.

Amethocaine is an alternative to EMLA® cream (a eutectic mixture of lidocaine and prilocaine) for skin anaesthesia not only in children but also in sensitive adults. Lignocaine is the drug of choice but it needs to be in gel formulation rather than aqueous liquid to hold to the urethral membrane and catheter during insertion. Lidocaine gel with adrenaline to reduce mucosal blood flow and hence mucosal volume has been used for preparation of the nose for intubation such as with nasogastric tubes but the use of a vasoconstrictor in the urethra is not required. Xylocaine spray is routinely used for throat mucosal anaesthesia typically used in upper GI endoscopy procedures.

8. B ★ OH Clin Surg, 4th edn → p211

Always check that a catheter is not blocked first by flushing it with some saline. If the catheter flushes freely but no urine is returned in the next 15min then there is acute oligoanuria present and the patient needs to be managed as for causes of that and a fluid bolus IV may then be correct. A bladder scan is not always accurate at determining if there is urine present and shouldn't be relied upon. If the flush fails then insertion of a new catheter may be appropriate but in this situation where there has been recent lower urinary tract surgery this should only be attempted by a senior with experience. Most importantly do not ignore it even if the patient is asymptomatic since the underlying diagnosis is important.

9. A ★★ OH Clin Surg, 4th edn → p190

The rhythm shown is ventricular tachycardia. Both pulseless ventricular tachycardia and ventricular fibrillation are shockable rhythms thus once identified the patient should be shocked without any delay and the ALS algorithm followed.

Adrenaline forms part of the ALS algorithm but has no direct effect on the cardiac rhythm.

Adenosine affects the atrioventricular nodal tissue to briefly prevent conduction and is used to break the cycle of re-entry tachycardias such as supraventricular tachycardia with or without bundle branch block but is only used in the presence of spontaneously maintained cardiac output (pulse present).

Amiodarone forms part of the ALS algorithm for tachycardia with a pulse present and is also used for less acute atrial fibrillation control.

lidocaine is no longer used in the resuscitation algorithms for acute membrane stabilization.

→ http://www.resus.org.uk/pages/alsalgo.pdf

10. D ★   OH Clin Surg, 4th edn → p217

Rigid sigmoidoscopy is done in outpatents without any sedation or medication. Bradycardia, induced by a high vagal response to colonic distension, can be experienced by some patients during intubation through the sigmoid colon such as during flexible sigmoidoscopy or colonoscopy but a rigid sigmoidoscopy, despite its name, does not pass through the sigmoid, only up to the top of the rectum. Perforation of the caecum is a risk of colonoscopy (quoted as around 1 in 1000 although the rate varies greatly depending on patient and colonic factors).

Rigid sigmoidoscopy puts hardly any stress on the normal anal muscular structures and damage leading to reduced continence is exceptionally unlikely but the scope may traumatize fragile anal canal lining tissues such as fissures or haemorrhoids and provoke some bleeding even if no other procedures are performed.

Extended Matching Questions

1. J ★

The increased systemic peripheral perfusion with low blood pressure and a tachycardia all point to a hyperdynamic circulation usually associated with infection. The swinging fever is typical of line sepsis but it could be arising from any site in the body and a full septic screen is necessary.

2. H ★

The rapid deterioration and shortness of breath indicate a complication affecting the respiratory or cardiovascular systems. The loss of breath sounds on the same side of the procedure indicates loss of lung expansion and the dullness makes it much more likely to be fluid accumulating in the pleura rather than air. The only fluid which will accumulate over 30min is blood making the diagnosis very likely to be a haemothorax (possibly from jugular vein laceration or more likely an incidental arterial injury during insertion).

3. F ★★

Cardiac tamponade is a recognized complication of central venous access usually due to atrial wall erosion or injury. It classically presents with three signs known as Beck's triad and these are: low arterial blood pressure, jugular venous distension, and muffled heart sounds. The ECG findings are typical of any fluid in the pericardium (blood or serous fluid).

4. E ★

Although neurological signs may develop in the presence of a venous thrombosis of the proximal limb vessels, they are usually slower in onset and associated with other changes. The cause of the acute neurology is often not direct needle injury but a haematoma in or immediately adjacent to the nerve causing pressure.

5. A ★★★

Venous air embolism is a predominantly iatrogenic complication that occurs when atmospheric gas is introduced into the systemic venous system. It has been associated with central venous catheterization, penetrating and blunt chest trauma, high-pressure mechanical ventilation, and other invasive vascular procedures. The general features present here are of a cardiovascular or respiratory complication but there are no lateral signs in the chest making pneumothorax and haemothorax unlikely. Because of the lack of specific signs and symptoms a high index of suspicion is necessary to establish the diagnosis and institute the appropriate treatment (a 'peri-arrest' call is required).

General feedback on 1–5:   OH Clin Surg, 4th edn → p198

Central line complications can be divided into:

Immediate: carotid artery puncture, pneumothorax, haemothorax, chylothorax, brachial plexus injury, arrhythmias, air embolism, and loss of guidewire into the right side of the heart.

Late: sepsis, thromboembolism, and arteriovenous fistula formation.

---

6. G ★★

Both these drugs require central venous administration to reduce the risk of toxicity. A rapidly available central venous catheter is required. It is unlikely to be needed in the longer term so there is no necessity for a tunnelled subclavian line. An internal jugular approach is often the easiest. With the history of carotid surgery most would favour a central approach via the heads of sternocleidomastoid rather than an anterior approach due to possible scarring and tethering of structures.

7. H ★   OH Clin Surg, 4th edn → p198

There are two options for this line; a peripherally inserted central catheter which is most commonly placed via the antecubital veins, not the brachial veins, and placed into the subclavian vein, or a tunnelled central venous catheter via the subclavian vein lying in the superior vena cava. Internal jugular central venous catheters are more susceptible to infective complications and not used for this length of time. The catheter used is usually tunnelled under the anterior chest wall skin to reduce the risk of line sepsis, one variety of which is referred to as a Hickman line.

8. C ★   OH Clin Surg, 4th edn → p200

Chest drains are best inserted well away from the vital structures of the chest. In the resuscitation room, a needle drain can be used in the anterior pleural space via the 3rd/4th intercostal space but this is a resuscitative manoeuvre for tension pneumothorax and can only safely be attempted with a needle and fine catheter. A formal chest drain which may be required for both air leak and blood/fluid removal should be inserted laterally where there is less chance of injury to vital structures.

9. D ★★   OH Clin Surg, 4th edn → p204

The best access to the pericardium is via its inferiormost extent which is furthest from the great vessels and easiest to access since it lies just deep to the sternal attachments of the diaphragm which can be passed through just below the xiphoid process. A parasternal approach risks injury to the internal thoracic artery or the great vessels and an approach over the ventricles of the heart risks injury to the lingula lobe of the lung and the pleura.

10. I ★★   OH Clin Surg, 4th edn → p198

Six weeks of treatment indicates the need for a central venous catheter. Although a subclavian venous approach is possible and does offer lower-risk sepsis in truly long-term catheters, a conventional internal jugular catheter with silver coating is perfectly adequate with a low risk of line sepsis and easier insertion and removal. Any approach is reasonable, such as the central one described here.

Chapter 4

Head and neck surgery

Gemma Conn

In almost no other surgical specialty does use of a diagnostic screen have such prominence than when considering the diagnosis of a lump in the head or neck. Is the lump neoplastic and if so, is it likely to be of benign, malignant, or of mixed malignant potential? Does the mass have features of a developmental condition or could it represent sequelae of acute or chronic infection? Are there associated signs suggesting endocrine or metabolic dysfunction in association with the mass? Is there a traumatic origin or are there features of degenerative disease?

Enlarged lymph nodes may be reactive due to inflammation, acute or chronic infection, or may represent primary or secondary neoplastic disease. Anatomical knowledge of lymph drainage patterns provides clues as to the region of primary pathology.

Developmental abnormalities such as thyroglossal cyst, dermoid inclusion cyst, and brachial fistula exhibit specific clinical signs and are found in characteristic anatomical locations.

Systemic clinical signs may occur in endocrine abnormalities associated with hyper- or hypothyroidism and, for instance, in primary hyperparathyroidism.

Bimanual examination will assist localization of sialolithiasis and the alert examiner will search for clinical involvement of the facial nerve which may help to suggest the nature of the neoplastic pathology involving a pre-auricular mass.

CT scan and fibre-endoscopy are powerful diagnostic tools in investigation of the oro- and nasopharynx and of the pathologies that may lie therein.

Head and neck pathologies may be treated by ENT, head & neck, or general surgical specialists. Irrespective of which specialty eventually manages the patient, it behoves the medical student and surgical trainee to ensure that he or she is conversant with the common clinical manifestations and anatomical features of conditions that occur in this region. This chapter will help you to revise distinct features of some of the most common clinical pathologies affecting the head and neck, and should remind you of rationales for specific diagnostic and therapeutic avenues.

Frank Smith

QUESTIONS

Single Best Answer

1. A 70-year-old farmer has a 0.5cm non-healing ulcer on his lower lip and a firm lump beneath his mandible. He sought medical advice reluctantly and cannot remember how long the lesions have been present. He is a pipe-smoker. Which is the *single* most likely diagnosis? ★

A Adenocarcinoma

B Actinomycosis

C Brucellosis

D Crohn's disease

E Squamous cell carcinoma

2. A 56-year-old man with no significant previous medical history develops a painless, progressively enlarging smooth mass anterior to his left ear. It has been slowly increasing in size for 3 months and is now 2cm in diameter. He has normal facial sensation and movements. Which is the *single* most likely diagnosis? ★★

A Adenocarcinoma

B Adenoid cystic carcinoma

C Adenolymphoma

D Mucoepidermoid tumour

E Pleomorphic adenoma

3. A 70-year-old man has facial pain and a lump anterior to his right ear. He has partial paralysis of facial muscles on the right side. His symptoms have developed over 2 years. The lump grew very slowly for most of that time but has increased in size significantly in the past 4 weeks and is now 3cm in diameter. Which is the *single* most likely diagnosis? ★★★

A Acinic cell carcinoma

B Adenoid cystic carcinoma

C Adenolymphoma

D Mucoepidermoid tumour

E Pleomorphic adenoma

4. A 50-year-old woman with type 1 diabetes has bilateral parotid swelling for 2 months. The parotid glands have doubled in size, are not tender, and are soft on palpation. She has no other symptoms. Which is the *single* most likely diagnosis? ★★★★

A Acute viral parotitis

B HIV parotitis

C Mikulicz disease

D Sialosis

E Sjögren's syndrome

5. A 40-year-old man has a tender lump beneath his left jawline. He has a year-long history of intermittent swelling and pain in this region on eating and drinking, although the pain has worsened in the past 3 days and has not been this severe before. The skin overlying it is red and warm to touch. He also has pain and muscle spasm on opening his jaw. His temperature is 38.2°C, pulse 86bpm, and blood pressure 127/78mmHg. Which is the *single* most likely diagnosis? ★★

A Acute sialadenitis

B Dental abscess

C Mucoepidermoid tumour

D Sialosis

E Sialolithiasis

6. A 30-year-old man has had a lump near the front of his neck for 18 months. It is visible anterior to the upper third of his sterno-cleidomastoid muscle. It recently rapidly increased in size, becoming tender, red, and warm to touch. However, following a course of antibiotics, the lump has returned to its usual size. Which is the *single* most likely diagnosis? ★

A Branchial cyst

B Cervical lymphadenopathy

C Cystic hygroma

D Sternocleidomastoid tumour

E Thyroglossal cyst

7. An 18-year-old student has had bilateral parotid swelling, testicular swelling, and general malaise for 1 week. Which is the *single* most likely causative organism? ★

A Adenovirus

B Cytomegalovirus

C Epstein–Barr virus

D Paramyxovirus

E Varicella zoster virus

8. A 38-year-old woman has a painless lump on the left side of her face. It has been present for 2 months. She has hypertension and fibromyalgia. An ultrasound scan reports an enlarged left parotid gland. She is on several medications. Which *single* drug is most likely to cause her symptoms? ★★★★

A Atenolol

B Bendroflumethiazide

C Co-dydramol

D Diltiazem

E Oral contraceptive pill

9. A 44-year-old woman with type 1 diabetes has an intermittent swelling beneath the right lower jaw on eating. A hard mass is palpable in the floor of her mouth. She first noticed her symptoms 1 year ago. Which is the *single* most likely diagnosis? ★

A Cervical lymphadenopathy

B Lymphoma

C Salivary gland adenocarcinoma

D Sialolithiasis

E Squamous cell carcinoma mouth

10. A 50-year-old woman has had painless bilateral swellings in her cheeks for 6 months. She also has several painful joints and mentions that her mouth always feels dry. Which is the *single* most likely diagnosis? ★

A Pleomorphic adenoma

B Sialolithiasis

C Sjögren's syndrome

D Tuberculosis

E Viral parotitis

11. A 24-year-old man has a 2cm lump in the middle of his neck that moves upwards on swallowing and on protrusion of the tongue. Which is the *single* most likely diagnosis? ★

A Branchial cyst

B Cervical lymphadenopathy

C Cystic hygroma

D Thyroid nodule

E Thyroglossal cyst

12. A 22-year-old engineering student has a swelling on the side of his neck which has enlarged over 4 days. It is visible at the anterior border of the sternomastoid muscle. There is localized erythema and tenderness. The lump is not fluctuant and he feels well in himself. His temperature is 36.9°C, pulse is 68bpm, and blood pressure 110/68mmHg. An ultrasound scan indicates that the swelling is cystic. Which is the *single* most appropriate initial management? ★

A Antibiotics

B Incision and drainage

C Needle aspiration

D NSAIDs

E Surgical excision

ANSWERS

Single Best Answers

1. E ★   OH Clin Surg, 4th edn → pp232–3

Squamous cell carcinoma is the most common tumour of the lips and oropharynx and sunlight and tobacco use are both risk factors. Other risk factors include male sex, high alcohol intake, poor oral hygiene, repeated trauma, e.g. ill-fitting dentures, infections including syphilis and human papillomavirus. Common presentations include non-healing ulcer, persistent sore throat, dysphagia, ear pain, odynophagia, and a palpable lump. Metastasis occurs to local lymph nodes. All levels of neck nodes should be examined. Adenocarcinoma is much less common.

Brucellosis is associated with occupations involving livestock handling such as farming, but would not present with a lip lesion as described.

Actinomycosis does present with facial and cervical swelling. Sinus tracts can develop between lesions and skin. This is not present in the scenario however.

Although Crohn's disease can cause ulceration anywhere along the GI tract, the rest of the history does not fit this diagnosis.

2. E ★★   OH Clin Surg, 4th edn → pp230–1

Pleomorphic adenomas occur most commonly in the 5th decade, with an equal sex distribution. They account for up to 80% of benign parotid gland tumours. They usually present as a painless, smooth enlarging mass. The facial nerve is not involved. Treatment by superficial parotidectomy is designed to spare the facial nerve, which is found in the plane between the superficial and deep parotid gland.

Mucoepidermoid tumour can present in a similar way but is less common than pleomorphic adenoma. They may grow slowly initially, with a period of accelerated growth before presentation.

Adenoid cystic carcinomas are relatively rare. They are more likely to cause symptoms in adjacent nerves.

Adenolymphoma, also known as Warthin's tumour, is the second most common parotid tumour. It is a possible diagnosis but tends to affect patients above 60 years of age.

Adenocarcinoma is a possible diagnosis but is less likely than the correct answer.

3. B ★★★   OH Clin Surg, 4th edn → p230

Acinic cell carcinoma is slow growing, rarely involves the facial nerve, but may occasionally metastasize unexpectedly.

Adenolymphoma is a benign soft swelling.

Adenoid cystic carcinoma is a tumour of the salivary glands. It is slow growing but may enlarge in spurts of growth. It often spreads along nerve sheaths resulting in facial pain and facial nerve palsy. Metastasis to lymph nodes is uncommon. Lung is the most common site of metastasis.

Mucoepidermoid tumours have low-grade malignancy, grow slowly, but may occasionally metastasize to lymph nodes, lung, and skin.

Pleomorphic adenoma is a tumour with low malignant potential which does not characteristically involve the facial nerve.

4. D ★★★★   OH Clin Surg, 4th edn → p230

Sialosis is recurrent swelling of the parotid gland that is usually soft, painless, and bilateral. It is associated with some drugs, metabolic and endocrine disorders. Sexes are affected equally, age of onset is generally between 20 and 60.

Parotitis is inflammation of the parotid glands which may occur in association with certain viral infections including HIV and paramyxovirus (mumps).

Sjögren's syndrome is an autoimmune disorder characterized by eye symptoms combined with rheumatoid arthritis or other connective tissue disorder.

Mikulicz disease is an autoimmune disorder and a variant of Sjögren's syndrome. It is characterized by the triad of enlargement of all salivary glands, enlargement of lacrimal glands (causing narrowed palpebral fissures), and dry mouth.

5. A ★★   OH Clin Surg, 4th edn → pp226–7

The submandibular gland duct lies below the mandible. Swelling in the submandibular gland is most commonly due to calculi, whereas in the parotid gland it is more commonly due to neoplasia. Stones may cause intermittent obstruction resulting in episodes of pain and swelling.

Acute suppurative sialadenitis is associated with fever and severe pain which may result in trismus or spasm of the muscles of mastication.

Sialosis refers to swelling of the salivary glands.

Sialithiasis refers to the presence of calculi in the duct.

6. A ★   OH Clin Surg, 4th edn → pp224–6

Branchial cysts are thought to be remnants of the 2nd and 3rd branchial arch. They may present at any age but are most common in the 3rd decade; 60–70% occur anteriorly to the upper border of sternocleidomastoid. The cyst may transilluminate on examination. Fine-needle aspiration cytology may contain cholesterol crystals, visible on microscopic examination. Branchial cysts may become infected resulting in an increase in size, with associated tenderness and erythema. This usually resolves with antibiotics, however, sometimes an abscess may develop requiring surgical drainage.

Cystic hygroma is a rare, benign lymphangioma of the neck.

Sternocleidomastoid tumour is the end result of muscle necrosis secondary to trauma (usually as a result of obstetric delivery). It presents as a hard lump in the muscle in the neonatal period and is associated with torticollis.

A thyroglossal cyst characteristically occurs in the midline, along the path of the thyroglossal duct and may demonstrate upward movement on tongue protrusion.

7. D ★   OH Clin Surg, 4th edn → pp228–9

Mumps is caused by the paramyxovirus which is a relative of the measles virus. Salivary gland inflammation results in jaw and face swelling. Symptoms include muscle pain, headache, low-grade pyrexia, malaise, earache, and difficulty in swallowing. Post puberty it may result in testicular inflammation which leads to pain and swelling. This may result in subfertility.

Adenoviruses cause a range of symptoms, most commonly respiratory. They can also cause general malaise, pharyngitis, conjunctivitis, fever, and lymphadenopathy.

Cytomegaloviruses are herpes viruses and a large proportion of the population has antibodies to them. Infections are usually subclinical or mild but can be more significant if the patient is immunosuppressed.

Epstein–Barr virus is a herpes virus and causes infectious mononucleosis (glandular fever). It is also associated with certain forms of cancer, including Burkitt's lymphoma and Hodgkin's lymphoma.

Varicella zoster virus is a herpesvirus that causes chickenpox and shingles.

8. E ★★★★

Drug-induced sialomegaly can be caused by medications including the oral contraceptive pill, thiouracil, co-proxamol, isoprenaline, and phenylbutazone.

9. D ★   OH Clin Surg, 4th edn → pp226–7

Salivary calculi typically present with intermittent pain and swelling on eating. Predisposing factors include reduced salivary flow, dehydration, duct obstruction, and chronic sialadenitis.

The submandibular duct runs from the submandibular gland (see Figure 4.1), which when enlarged is palpable, to its opening at the base of the tongue. An impacted stone may be palpable on bimanual examination which should form part of the clinical examination.

Certain medical conditions predispose to sialolithiasis, including diabetes, liver disease, and hypertension.

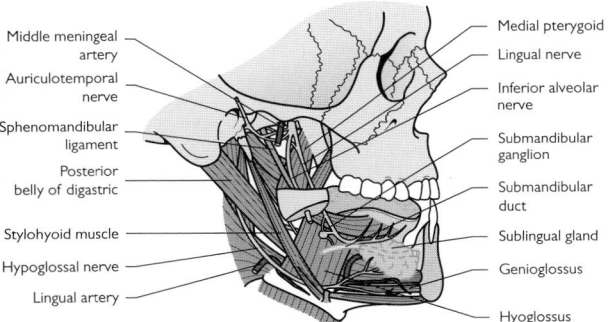

Figure 4.1 The submandibular gland and surrounding anatomical structures

Reproduced from Atkinson, *Anatomy for Dental Students*, 4th edition, 2013, with permission from Oxford University Press.

---

10. C ★   OH Clin Surg, 4th edn → pp228–9

Sjögren's syndrome is an autoimmune condition characterized by dry eyes (keratoconjunctivitis sicca), xerostomia, and connective tissue disorders such as rheumatoid arthritis, scleroderma, or systemic lupus erythematosus.

Pleomorphic adenoma is a benign parotid gland tumour. They would not be associated with the other mentioned symptoms.

Sialolithiasis—the formation of stones in the salivary glands—similarly would have symptoms related to those structures.

Viral parotitis (mumps) does involve glandular swelling, but otherwise the clinical picture is not as described.

Tuberculosis can present in many different ways, but the set of symptoms in the question is much more indicative of Sjögren's disease.

---

11. E ★   OH Clin Surg, 4th edn → pp222–3

The thyroid gland descends from the base of the tongue to its definitive anatomical position during embryological development. The persistence of a segment of this tract can result in a thyroglossal cyst. This presents as a midline swelling that moves upwards on swallowing and protrusion of the tongue, due to attachment of the cord of cells forming the duct remnant, to the foramen caecum at the dorsal surface of the tongue (see Figure 4.2). A thyroid mass will move upward on swallowing but it is the movement on tongue protrusion that differentiates the thyroglossal cyst clinically from other lesions, including cystic hygroma and branchial cyst.

A thyroglossal cyst is differentiated from ectopic thyroid tissue by ultrasound, CT, or isotope scan.

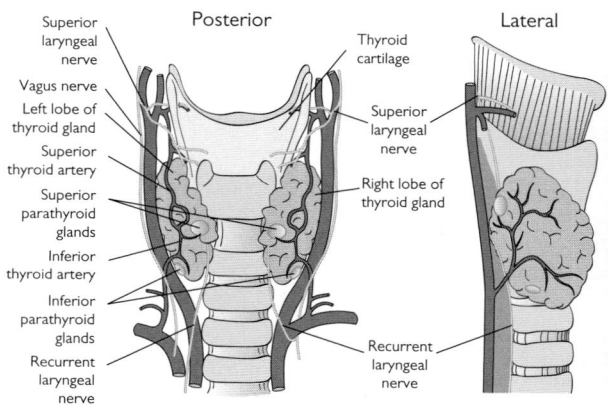

Figure 4.2 The position of the thyroid gland
Reproduced from Longmore et al., *Oxford Handbook of Clinical Medicine*, 7th edition, 2007, with permission from Oxford University Press.

12. A ★ OH Clin Surg, 4th edn → pp224–5

A simple infected branchial cyst without signs of systemic infection or abscess formation should respond to antibiotics. Surgical drainage or aspiration is not indicated initially, and the infection should be treated first.

If an abscess forms, usually indicated by an enlarging, erythematous, fluctuant swelling, then an incision and drainage should be performed.

The patient may then have an elective surgical excision at a later date.

Chapter 5

Breast and endocrine surgery

Asmaa Al-Alaak

One of the main 'complaints' about breast disease is that 'it is all so similar' and that there are lots of treatment options which can seem confusing at first. The key to understanding breast disease and preparing for questions about it is to keep the basic facts about breast anatomy and pathology to the forefront, learn to recognize key patterns of clinical signs and symptoms, and then match them to the clinical scenario. The EMQs are particularly useful at practising fitting questions into clinical patterns and rehearsing the patterns.

Endocrine disease poses its own challenges. Even for a surgeon it is important to understand and recognize the underlying biochemistry and how this affects the clinical presentations. Endocrine surgical disease is much less about anatomy or surgical procedures themselves as it is about understanding how treatment is matched to the pathophysiology of the conditions.

Neil Borley

QUESTIONS

Single Best Answers

1. A 40-year-old woman has had 3 weeks of unilateral breast pain. The pain has been constant with no relation to her menstrual cycle. She has a past medical history of asthma with a recent episode of exacerbation. There is no evidence of any discrete lumps or axillary lymphadenopathy. There is localized tenderness on palpation of the medial half of the left breast and over the 4th and 5th costochondral junctions. Which is the *single* most likely diagnosis? ★

A Atypical angina

B Breast abscess

C Cyclical mastalgia

D Mastitis

E Tietze's syndrome

2. A 35-year-old woman has been recently diagnosed by her GP with Graves' disease and has been referred to the outpatient department for further management. She has no other past medical history. She is a housewife and looks after her three young children aged 1 to 6. She has a large goitre with signs of severe exophthalmos (see Figure 5.1).

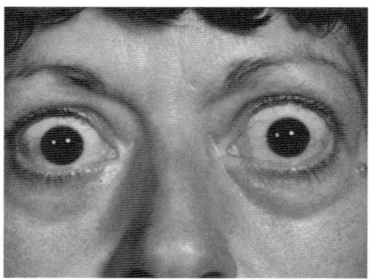

Figure 5.1 Exophthalmos
Reproduced from Longmore et al., *Oxford Handbook of Clinical Medicine*, 8th edition, 2010, with permission from Oxford University Press.

Which is the *single* most appropriate long term treatment option for this lady? ★★★

A Carbimazole 20mg twice a day

B Propylthiouracil 200mg twice a day

C Radioactive iodine

D Subtotal thyroidectomy

E Thyroid lobectomy

3. A 50-year-old woman has had intermittent nipple discharge. She has noticed that the discharge seems to be coming from one point on the left nipple. The discharge is slightly blood-stained. There are no discrete lumps and no axillary lymphadenopathy. On gentle squeezing of the left nipple there is a single point of discharge. A mammogram is normal. Which is the *single* most likely diagnosis? ★

A Acute suppurative mastitis

B Duct papilloma

C Duct ectasia

D Fibrocystic disease

E Periductal mastitis

4. A 50-year-old woman has had 3 weeks of pain in front of her neck. She also complains of general malaise, episodes of feeling feverish, and palpitations. She has no past medical history and is not on any regular medications. She has a diffusely tender, slightly enlarged thyroid gland. Which is the *single* most likely diagnosis? ★★★

A De Quervain's thyroiditis

B Graves' disease

C Hashimoto's thyroiditis

D Physiological thyroid enlargement

E Thyroid papillary carcinoma

5. A 90-year-old woman has a swelling in her neck which has increased in size over the last 2 weeks. She reports difficulty in swallowing, shortness of breath, coughing, and a hoarse voice. She has a large fixed mass in the left anterior triangle of her neck with palpable cervical lymphadenopathy. Which is the *single* most likely diagnosis? ★

A Anaplastic cancer

B Follicular cancer

C Lymphoma

D Medullary cancer

E Papillary cancer

6. A 35-year-old woman has had a painful lump in her neck for 1 month. She has no other related symptoms. She has a solitary thyroid nodule that is slightly tender. A fine-needle aspiration biopsy (FNAB) gives a result of Thy2. Which is the *single* most likely diagnosis? ★

A Benign colloid nodule

B Follicular lesion

C Graves' disease

D Medullary carcinoma of the thyroid

E Normal thyroid

7. A 40-year-old woman has undergone a total thyroidectomy for a multinodular goitre. She is a member of her local choir and has noticed that she is no longer able to reach high notes as she used to prior to her surgery and that her voice fatigues. Which is the *single* most likely nerve that has been injured at surgery? ★★★★

A External laryngeal nerve

B Glossopharyngeal nerve

C Internal laryngeal nerve

D Recurrent laryngeal nerve

E Ansa cervicalis

8. Figure 5.2 is a graphic illustration of the formation of various thyroid hormones by thyroid epithelial cells. I⁻ is ionic iodine, del indicates the process of de-iodinization, and AA circulating amino acids. Four structurally different hormones are indicated by the letters W, X, Y, and Z.

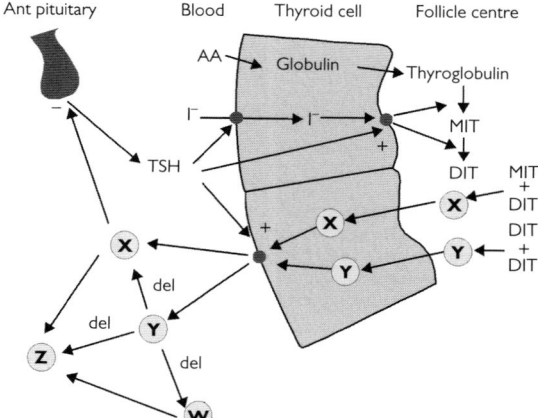

Figure 5.2 The formation of various thyroid hormones by thyroid epithelial cells

Which is the *single* correct name of the hormone X? ★

A Di-iodothyronine

B Di-iodotyrosine

C Reverse tri-iodothyronine

D Thyroxine

E Tri-iodothyronine

9. A 57-year-old woman has noticed a lump in the right breast for 4 weeks. She is otherwise fit and well and is not on any regular medications. On triple assessment she is found to have two foci of invasive ductal carcinoma with widespread ductal carcinoma *in situ* and FNAB of enlarged axillary lymph nodes confirms tumour involvement. Which is the *single* most appropriate surgical treatment for this patient? ★

A Mastectomy and axillary node clearance

B Mastectomy and radiotherapy

C Mastectomy and sentinel node biopsy

D Wide local excision and axillary node clearance

E Wide local excision and sentinel node biopsy

10. A 40-year-old premenopausal woman has recently been diagnosed with breast cancer. She has had a wide local excision and sentinel node biopsy. Histology of the tumour reveals a 1.8cm grade 2 invasive ductal carcinoma which is oestrogen receptor positive. The sentinel node did not contain tumour. Which is the *single* most appropriate hormonal treatment for this patient? ★★★

A Anastrazole

B Letrozole

C None

D Tamoxifen

E Goserelin

11. A 70-year-old woman has had a lump in her left breast for 12 months. This lump has gradually increased in size and she has recently noticed that the shape of her breast has changed. She denies any other symptoms. She has evidence of skin dimpling in the outer aspect of the left breast and has a hard fixed mass with palpable axillary lymph nodes. Which is the *single* most likely diagnosis? ★

A Breast cancer

B Fat necrosis

C Fibrocystic disease

D Mastitis

E Surgical scar

12. A 52-year-old woman has noticed 10 days of diffuse pain, redness, and swelling of the right breast. A course of antibiotics for the last 5 days has had no effect. Her nipple has changed shape with some associated discharge. A mammogram last year was normal but there is skin and subcutaneous oedema seen on ultrasound scan which is uncomfortable. Her breast is swollen, tender, and firm, as shown in Figure 5.3.

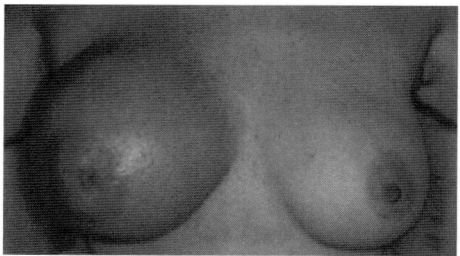

Figure 5.3 Her breast is swollen, tender, and firm
Reproduced with permission from UBM Media. See *Acknowledgements* for full details.

Which is the *single* most likely diagnosis? ★★

A Breast abscess

B Graves' disease

C Inflammatory breast cancer

D Insect bite

E Mastitis

13. A 40-year-old man has had 1 month of spontaneous episodes of palpitations, headaches, sweating, and chest pain lasting for up to 15min. A diagnosis of phaeochromocytoma is considered. Which is the *single* most appropriate initial investigation that will help to confirm the diagnosis? ★

A Aldosterone suppression test

B Clonidine suppression test

C Long synacthen test

D Short synacthen test

E 24h urine for vanillylmandelic acid and noradrenaline

14. A 65-year-old woman is referred by her GP following a routine blood test which showed a raised serum calcium. Over the last few months she has become constipated with intermittent bouts of abdominal pain. She is lethargic and her mood has been very low. Clinical examination is unremarkable. Biochemical results show a corrected serum calcium of 2.95mmol/L and a serum parathyroid hormone of 24pmol/L. Which is the *single* most likely diagnosis? ★

A Addison's disease

B Lymphoma

C 'Milk-alkali' syndrome

D Multiple myeloma

E Primary hyperparathyroidism

15. A 65-year-old man has recently gained a significant amount of weight, his hair has become very dry and brittle, and his mood is low. He has a round face with a prominent fat pad along his back. Which is the *single* most appropriate subsequent investigation? ★★

A Abdominal CT scan

B Abdominal MRI scan

C Dexamethasone suppression test

D Early morning cortisol level

E Pituitary MRI scan

Extended Matching Questions

Breast problems

For each scenario choose the *single* most likely diagnosis from the list of options. Each option may be used once, more than once, or not at all.

A Breast carcinoma

B Breast cyst

C Duct ectasia

D Fat necrosis

E Fibroadenoma

F Galactocoele

G Lactational mastitis

H Lipoma

I Periductal mastitis

1. A 20-year-old woman is seen in the breast clinic with a lump in her right breast for 1 month. She has a 1cm discrete, mobile lump in the lower outer quadrant of the right breast which is non-tender. ★

2. A 50-year-old woman has suffered a painful lump in the right breast for 3 weeks. Over the last few months she has had irregular periods and hot flushes. There is a 2cm discrete, moderately tender lump in the lower inner quadrant of her right breast with normal-looking breast skin. Ultrasound scan shows a well-defined lesion and needle aspiration yielded 12mL of a green-yellow fluid. ★

3. A 40-year-old woman has found an asymptomatic lump in the central portion of her right breast. Past medical history includes diabetes mellitus and a fractured collar bone in a road traffic collision 3 months ago. There is a semimobile irregular lump in the central portion of the right breast with overlying skin haemosiderin deposition. There is no evidence of axillary lymphadenopathy. ★★

4. A 32-year-old woman has had 5 weeks of redness and swelling around the right nipple. There is no past medical history but she is a heavy smoker. There is periareolar skin inflammation with a small palpable tender mass just behind the nipple. ★

5. A 60-year-old woman has noted that in the last few months both nipples have gradually retracted. She is also complaining of significant nipple discharge that is thick and yellow/green in colour. Both nipples are retracted and slit-like with no palpable lumps or lymphadenopathy. ★★★★

Breast lumps

For each scenario choose the *single* most appropriate next treatment from the list of options. Each option may be used once, more than once, or not at all.

A Anastrozole

B Excision biopsy

C External beam radiotherapy

D Neoadjuvant chemotherapy

E Mastectomy and sentinel node biopsy

F Mastectomy and axillary node clearance

G Tamoxifen

H Trastuzumab

I Wire-guided wide local excision

J Wide local excision and sentinel node biopsy

K Wide local excision and axillary node clearance

6. An 84-year-old woman presents with a 2-month history of a lump in her left breast. She has a past medical history of ischaemic heart disease and previous deep vein thrombosis. She has a very limited exercise tolerance with shortness of breath on minimal exertion. Triple assessment reveals a grade 2 invasive ductal carcinoma which is oestrogen receptor positive. ★★★★

7. A 50-year-old woman is diagnosed with a small area of microcalcification in the left breast measuring approximately 12mm under the national breast cancer screening programme. Stereotactic core biopsies confirm the presence of low-grade ductal carcinoma *in situ*. ★★

8. A 60-year-old woman is diagnosed with a palpable invasive ductal carcinoma. She undergoes a wide local excision and sentinel node biopsy. Histology confirms the presence of a 10mm grade 1 invasive ductal carcinoma which is completely excised with no evidence of lymph node involvement. The tumour is oestrogen receptor negative. ★★

9. An 82-year-old woman is 3 years post mastectomy and axillary node clearance for a lymph node positive, grade 3 breast cancer. She has developed proven spinal metastases on bone scanning which are causing back pain but there is no threat to her spinal cord from compression. ★★

10. A 32-year-old woman presents with a 3-month history of a large lump in the right breast. There is an 8cm diameter mass and palpable axillary lymphadenopathy. Core biopsy of the lump confirms invasive ductal carcinoma and FNAB of the axillary nodes is positive for carcinoma. ★★★★

Neck lumps

For each scenario choose the *single* most likely diagnosis from the list of options. Each option may be used once, more than once, or not at all.

A Branchial cyst

B Cervical rib

C Chemodectoma

D Cystic hygroma

E Lipoma

F Lymphoma

G Thyroid tumour

H Sebaceous cyst

I Thyroglossal cyst

11. A 30-year-old man has had a lump on the right side of his neck for a number of years which intermittently discharges. There is a discrete lump in the posterior triangle of the neck which is superficial, mobile, and has a visible punctum. ★

12. A 20-year-old man has an asymptomatic swelling just to the right side of the midline of the anterior neck. It feels firm and moves on protrusion of the tongue. ★

13. A 15-year-old boy attends the outpatient department with his mother. She has noticed a lump in his neck over the last few months. This occasionally increases in size causing pain and discomfort. The child has a smooth, non-tender, fluctuant mass along the lower anteromedial border of sternocleidomastoid. ★★

14. A 50-year-old man has noticed a lump in his neck which has slightly increased in size over the last few months. There is a soft, mobile, non-tender lump in the left anterior triangle of the neck and several smaller, similar lumps in both triangles of the right side of the neck. ★

15. A 35-year-old woman is seen in the clinic with an enlarging left-sided neck swelling. She has lost 9kg over the last 4 weeks and has become very lethargic. There is a diffuse, rubbery, firm feeling mass in the left anterior triangle with associated palpable cervical and axillary lymphadenopathy. ★

Treating endocrine disorders

For each scenario choose the *single* most appropriate next line of treatment from the list of options. Each option may be used once, more than once, or not at all.

A Bromocriptine 1.25–2.5mg once daily

B Carbimazole 40mg once daily

C Digoxin 125mcg once daily

D Furosemide 40mg

E Levothyroxine 20mcg three times daily

F Thyroxine 100–200mcg once daily

G Thyroxine 25–100mcg once daily

H Pamidronate 90mg intravenously

I Propranolol 40mg once daily

J Propylthiouracil 30mg once daily

K Spironolactone 50–100mg once daily

16. A 68-year-old woman attends pre-admission clinic prior to her surgery for a parathyroid adenoma. She has some routine blood tests at the time and her corrected calcium is 3.2mmol/L. She is admitted before her surgery and is rehydrated aggressively but a repeat corrected calcium remains at 3.02mmol/L. ★★★★

17. A 58-year-old man presents with symptoms of muscle weakness, cramping, intermittent paralysis, and headaches. He has also noticed that he is always thirsty and is getting up frequently at night to pass urine. He has a blood pressure of 205/110mmHg and K^+ of 2.8mmol/L. A CT scan of his abdomen shows a solitary mass in the right adrenal gland. ★★★

18. A 37-year-old woman has been recently diagnosed with a papillary carcinoma of the thyroid. She has undergone a total thyroidectomy as part of her initial treatment. ★★★

19. A 32-year-old woman has lost a significant amount of weight over the last few months even though her appetite has been normal. She has had a few episodes of palpitations and has a noticeable hand tremor. She has a noticeable tremor, her palms are sweaty and her heart rate is 120bpm. Her thyroid stimulating hormone (TSH) is 0.2mU/L and thyroxine (T_4) is 201nmol/L. ★

20. A 60-year-old woman has just undergone a total thyroidectomy for cancer of the thyroid gland. As part of her postoperative treatment plan she will undergo a ^{131}I-whole body scan. ★★

ANSWERS

Single Best Answers

1. E ★

OH Clin Surg, 4th edn → p248

Breast pain is a common symptom reported by women attending breast clinics. Most cases are minor and accepted as part of the normal changes that occur in relation to the menstrual cycle. In this scenario the most likely cause of the pain is Tietze's syndrome, caused by an inflammatory process arising in one or more of the costal cartilages. It is usually short-lived and self-limiting but may also become a chronic condition. It may result from a strain or minor injury, such as coughing, sneezing, vomiting, or hard repetitive exercise. NSAIDs help in the management of pain.

2. D ★★★

OH Clin Surg, 4th edn → p253

Medical therapy is often effective and is the usual first-line treatment in Graves' disease but not in this lady. Radioiodine is contraindicated with her age and young children. In cases of severe eye signs, the risk of permanent damage usually indicates proceeding directly to surgery to control the disease quickly. Indications for subtotal thyroidectomy include cancer, benign multinodular goitre when both lobes are involved with significant nodules, toxic multinodular goitre, and Graves' disease. It is also indicated in patients whose symptoms have been difficult to control on medication. Subtotal thyroidectomy can be done safely with a low rate of complications. The incidence of permanent recurrent laryngeal nerve injury and permanent hypoparathyroidism is <1%. In this case the patient has a young family thus treatment with radioactive iodine is not an option.

→ http://www.springerlink.com/content/bkuylwtntua56mmm/fulltext.pdf

3. B ★

OH Clin Surg, 4th edn → p246

Ductal papillomas occur within large, central mammary lactiferous ducts. They are epithelial proliferations which may occur singly or as part of a syndrome of multiple intraductal papillomatosis. There is an increased risk of malignancy associated with multiple papillomata. It is commonest in premenopausal women and presents with nipple discharge and small-volume bleeding. Differential diagnoses include Paget's disease, adenoma of the nipple, and carcinoma. Mammography is indicated. Surgical treatment is by excision of the affected area of breast tissue—microdochectomy.

4. A ★★★

OH Clin Surg, 4th edn → p252

The painful tender swelling of the thyroid is strongly suggestive of inflammation. It is uncommon in tumours and effectively excludes physiological enlargement. Graves' disease is less likely to cause a tender gland. Hashimoto's disease may cause a slightly swollen gland early in its course but more commonly the gland is shrunken and impalpable. It is the most common cause of a painful thyroid gland. Most patients have pain in the region of the thyroid, which is usually diffusely tender, and some have systemic symptoms. As is the case for most thyroid diseases, de Quervain's thyroiditis appears more frequently in females, with a female-to-male ratio of 3–5:1. The peak incidence is in the 4th and 5th decades of life. The natural course of the disease can be divided into the following four phases that usually unfold over a period of 3–6 months:

1. Acute phase: lasting 3–6 weeks, presents primarily with pain. Symptoms of hyperthyroidism may also be present.
2. Transient asymptomatic and euthyroid phase: lasts 1–3 weeks.
3. Hypothyroid phase: lasts from weeks to months, and may be permanent in 5–15% of patients.
4. Recovery phase: is characterized by normalization of thyroid structure and function.

5. A ★   OH Clin Surg, 4th edn → p256

The fixity of the mass and the associated lymphadenopathy make a primary malignancy of the thyroid very likely. The age of the patient and the fixity of the mass makes anaplastic carcinoma the most likely. Anaplastic carcinoma of the thyroid is the most aggressive thyroid gland malignancy. Although it accounts for <2% of all thyroid cancers, it causes up to 40% of deaths from thyroid cancer. It generally occurs in people in iodine-deficient areas and in a setting of previous thyroid pathology (pre-existing goitre, follicular thyroid cancer, papillary thyroid cancer). Local invasion of adjacent structures (trachea, oesophagus) commonly occurs. It has a rapid course and early dissemination. The most common sites of distant spread include the lungs, bone, and brain. Metastases, particularly in the lung, are likely to be present at diagnosis in >50% of cases.

6. A ★   OH Clin Surg, 4th edn → p256

FNAB is the initial investigation of choice for thyroid nodules. The cytology results are usually presented in a 5-point scale:

Thy 1: non-diagnostic sample
Thy 2: benign colloid nodule
Thy 3: follicular lesion
Thy 4: suspicious but not diagnostic
Thy 5: diagnostic for thyroid cancer.

Follicular neoplasms cannot be separated (invasive or non-invasive) on FNAB.

7. A ★★★★ OH Clin Surg, 4th edn → p268

The superior laryngeal nerve has two divisions: internal and external. The internal branch provides sensory innervation to the larynx. It enters the larynx through the thyrohyoid membrane and, therefore, should not be at risk during thyroidectomy. The external branch provides motor function to the cricothyroid muscle and is at risk during thyroidectomy. This muscle is involved in elongation of the vocal folds. Trauma to the nerve results in an inability to lengthen a vocal fold and, thus, an inability to create a high-pitched sound. The recurrent laryngeal nerve supplies the intrinsic laryngeal muscles and loss or reduced function of the nerve results in weakness or paralysis of the vocal cord on the affected side. If unilateral this leads to a husky voice and inability to cough normally due to failure to be able to close the larynx prior to air expulsion ('bovine cough'). The glossopharyngeal and ansa cervicalis (sympathetic) do not innervate either motor or sensory functions of the larynx but innervate the pharynx.

8. D ★ OH Clin Surg, 4th edn → p252

The thyroid gland produces many biochemically active compounds and two are normally released into the circulation although four compounds are present. Their biological activities are different and they exist both bound to proteins (mostly albumin) and free to varying extents. Di-iodotyrosine is the full name of DIT formed within the follicle and it is not normally released. Both thyroxine (T_4) (compound Y) and tri-iodothyronine (T_3) (compound X) are released although most T_3 comes from the reduction of thyroxine (T_4) in the peripheral circulation. Only thyroxine (T_4) is de-iodinated to form reverse tri-iodothyronine (rT_3) (compound W) which is *not* produced from the thyroid cells directly. Di-iodothyronine (T_2) is the inactive final reduction form of all three hormones only formed peripherally. The principle suppressor of TSH release is T_3 due to it having five times greater biological activity than T_4 and more than ten times greater activity than rT_3.

9. A ★ OH Clin Surg, 4th edn → p242

The most appropriate treatment in this case is a mastectomy given that there is evidence of multifocal widespread disease and axillary node clearance is indicated due to clinically pathological lymph nodes. If there had been no evidence of lymph node involvement then a mastectomy and sentinel node biopsy would have been the best option. Wide local excision of the breast is not an option in this case due to the risk of leaving other foci of microinvasive disease.

10. D ★★★ OH Clin Surg, 4th edn → p240

The most appropriate treatment for this lady is tamoxifen. Both anastrozole and letrozole are aromatase inhibitors that are mainly used in postmenopausal women since their main mechanism of action is to stop the production of oestrogen in peripheral tissue by inhibiting the effect of the enzyme aromatase. Aromatase inhibitors have no effect on ovarian production of oestrogen hence their use in postmenopausal women.

In some cases when young patients have a poor prognosis tumour aromatase inhibitors can be used in combination with goserelin, a gonadorelin analogue that suppresses the production of both luteinizing hormone (LH) and follicle-stimulating hormone (FSH) thus suppressing the production of oestrogen by the ovaries.

11. A ★ OH Clin Surg, 4th edn → p240

Skin dimpling or change in the contour of the breast is present in up to 40% of patients with breast cancer and is usually due to the tumour being close to the skin and may be a late presentation. The other listed options are all benign causes of skin dimpling. The fixity of the mass is most likely in breast cancer or fat necrosis. The presence of the lymphadenopathy is most suggestive of breast carcinoma.

12. C ★★ OH Clin Surg, 4th edn → p240

The most likely diagnosis in this case is inflammatory breast cancer. It is an especially aggressive type of breast cancer that can occur in women of any age. The rapid onset of symptoms is a feature and the clinical signs of swelling, erythema, and skin oedema can be misdiagnosed as mastitis. Many of the symptoms relate to impaired lymphatic drainage from the breast due to local invasion by tumour which can precipitate a sudden worsening of symptoms. The skin of the breast is relatively tethered by internal connective tissue septae ('ligaments of Cooper'), the oedema causes localized skin changes with dimpling resembling orange peel (peau d'orange). Inflammatory breast cancer can be misdiagnosed as an acute cause of infection such as a bite, tiny penetrating injury, or breast infection. A lump may well not be present or detectable but the diffuse nature of the inflammation is against this being an abscess. Acute severe mastitis would usually have responded to antibiotics to some degree.

Other typical symptoms of inflammatory breast cancer include itching of breast, nipple retraction or discharge, and palpable lymph nodes in the axilla and neck. The only reliable method of diagnosis is a biopsy.

13. E ★ OH Clin Surg, 4th edn → p268

Phaeochromocytomas produce a wide range of catecholamines including dopamine, adrenaline, and noradrenaline. The 24h urine collection for vanillylmandelic acid and noradrenaline is the most accurate investigation for the diagnosis of phaeochromocytoma with a 97% sensitivity. The clonidine suppression test is used when the results of urinary catecholamines are equivocal. Clonidine, a centrally acting alpha-adrenergic agonist, suppresses neurogenic-mediated catecholamines, and should not suppress the release of catecholamines from a phaeochromocytoma which is independent of normal control. The synacthen tests are used in the diagnosis of adrenocortical hormone abnormalities as is the aldosterone suppression test.

14. E ★ OH Clin Surg, 4th edn → p260

Primary hyperparathyroidism is the inappropriate secretion of parathyroid hormone to the level of circulating calcium. The main cause is usually due to a parathyroid adenoma. Its incidence is approximately 42 per 100 000 people and is three times as common in women than men. The signs and symptoms of primary hyperparathyroidism are those of hypercalcaemia. They are classically summarized by the mnemonic 'stones, bones, abdominal groans, and psychic moans'. Treatment is usually surgical with bilateral neck exploration and visualization of all four parathyroid glands.

15. C ★★ OH Clin Surg, 4th edn → p264

The clinical picture is classic of Cushing's syndrome. Other features might be brittle nails, skin thinning with easy bruising, and the development of striae. The obesity is classically abdominal/truncal with wasting of the limb muscles ('orange on sticks'). Mood changes can be variable and include psychosis in extreme cases. The first investigation of choice in this case is the dexamethasone suppression test in order to confirm the diagnosis of Cushing's syndrome. It is more reliable than measurement of the cortisol levels or the 24h cortisol excretion. Once the diagnosis is established then further investigations to determine the cause can be requested which might include CT or MRI scanning.

Extended Matching Questions

1. E ★ OH Clin Surg, 4th edn → p246

Fibroadenoma is a benign breast lump that is classified as an aberration of normal breast development. It is most commonly seen in young women under the age of 30. Typical features are that of a discrete, mobile, painless lump. They are usually solitary findings but some women develop multiple lesions in one or both breasts.

2. B ★ OH Clin Surg, 4th edn → p246

Breast cysts are benign breast lumps that are most common in perimenopausal women. They may be discrete or multiple and are usually tender. Diagnosis is usually confirmed on aspiration of a green-yellow fluid. It is very unlikely to be a galactocoele given that she is menopausal and a breast abscess would be likely to be much more tender with associated overlying changes.

3. D ★★   OH Clin Surg, 4th edn → p247

Fat necrosis may follow trauma to the breast. There may be no obvious history of trauma and there is considerable overlap with the features of malignancy on clinical examination. In this case the presence of haemosiderin deposition is evidence of a significant disruptive injury to the breast tissue and tumour necrosis factor is the most likely cause.

4. I ★

Periductal mastitis is most commonly seen in young women. Evidence suggests that smoking is an important factor in the aetiology of the disease. Initial presentation may be with periareolar inflammation (with or without an associated mass). Other features may be pain, nipple retraction, and nipple discharge.

5. C ★★★★

Duct ectasia is the dilatation and shortening of ducts during breast involution. When this process is excessive women present with a cheesy nipple discharge and nipple retraction which is classically slit-like. Surgery may be indicated in some cases when the discharge is troublesome. Unilateral nipple retraction may be a sign of underlying malignancy but it is almost always unilateral in that case.

6. A ★★★★

The most appropriate management for this patient is primary hormonal therapy since she is unlikely to tolerate a general anaesthetic. Anastrazole is the drug of choice in this case rather than tamoxifen given her past medical history of deep vein thrombosis.

7. I ★★

Excision biopsy is required in the first instance. Since this is a very small area of abnormality it is unlikely to be clinically palpable. Thus a wire is inserted to localise the lesion so that this can be surgically excised.

8. C ★★

Patients who undergo wide local excision for breast cancer require postoperative radiotherapy to reduce the risk of recurrence. This is the only treatment that this patient needs since it is a small tumour that is oestrogen receptor negative.

9. C ★★

Bone metastases may respond to many forms of treatment depending on their hormone receptor profile and chemosensitivity but external beam radiotherapy is an excellent quick treatment for the associated bone pain and can be supplemented with other treatment subsequently.

10. D ★★★★

The tumour will need to be excised and the axillary nodes completely dissected (clearance). It is unlikely that a wide local excision will be possible with the size of the tumour and although a mastectomy may well be effective for local excision neoadjuvant chemotherapy is the treatment of choice; it may down stage the tumour to allow the possibility of considering breast conservation surgery rather than more extensive surgery and has the theoretical advantage of treating potential micrometastases immediately in what is poor prognosis disease.

11. H ★

A sebaceous cyst is as a closed sac under the skin derived from the sebaceous glands of the skin and filled with the cheese-like, oily result of impacted gland secretions. They are extremely common and probably most people will have one over the course of a lifetime. Often they resolve spontaneously. They are said to be twice as common in men as in women and most frequent in the 20s and 30s. The presence of the central punctum is characteristic and the location in the posterior triangle makes other cystic masses of the neck unlikely.

12. I ★

Thyroglossal duct cysts most often present with a palpable asymptomatic neck mass below the level of the hyoid bone. Although they originate from a midline structure, as they enlarge they often lie just to one side or other of the midline. The mass moves during swallowing or on protrusion of the tongue because of its attachment to the tongue via the tract of thyroid descent. Up to half of thyroglossal cysts are not diagnosed until adult life. The tract can lie dormant for years or even decades until some kind of stimulus leads to cystic dilation. Infection can sometimes cause the transient appearance of a mass or enlargement of the cyst, at times with periodic recurrences. Spontaneous drainage may also occur. The cyst is often tense and hence can feel firm or even solid.

13. A ★★

Branchial cysts are congenital epithelial cysts, which arise on the lateral part of the neck from a failure of obliteration of the second branchial cleft in embryonic development. Although congenital in nature they may not present clinically until later in life, usually by early adulthood. They are smooth, nontender, fluctuant masses, which occur along the lower one third of the anteromedial border of the sternocleidomastoid muscle between the muscle and the overlying skin.

14. E ★

A lipoma is a benign tumour composed of fatty tissue. They are the most common form of soft tissue tumour. They are soft to the touch, usually movable, and are generally painless. The neck is a relatively common location. The presence of multiple lumps may be suggestive of benign lymphadenopathy or lymphoma but the length of history is against the former and lymphomatous nodes are usually matted or confluent.

15. F ★

Lymphoma is the most common form of haematological malignancy in the developed world. Taken together, lymphomas represent 5.3% of all cancers (excluding simple basal cell and squamous cell skin cancers) in the United States and 55.6% of all haematological malignancies. Symptoms include: anorexia, dyspnoea, fatigue, lymphadenopathy, night sweats, pruritus, and weight loss. The presence of the cervical and axillary lymphadenopathy is highly suggestive of lymphoma rather than a primary neck tumour.

16. D ★★★★   OH Clin Surg, 4th edn → p261

The most common cause of hypercalcaemia is primary hyperparathyroidism (PHPT). The treatment of choice is surgery but in cases where the corrected calcium is > 3mmol/L then aggressive rehydration is indicated first. If the levels remain high then the next option would be to try furosemide which increases urinary excretion of calcium. Bisphosphonates (such as pamidronate) should be avoided in PHPT when surgery is anticipated since they can impair the ability to maintain normal calcium levels following surgery.

17. K ★★★   OH Clin Surg, 4th edn → p266

Conn's syndrome is characterised by increased aldosterone secretion from the adrenal glands, suppressed plasma renin activity (PRA), hypertension, and hypokalaemia. It was first described in 1954 by JW Conn. Patients with severe hypokalaemia report fatigue, muscle weakness, cramping, headaches, and palpitations. They can also have polydipsia and polyuria from hypokalaemia-induced nephrogenic diabetes insipidus. Spironolactone can be used to control hypertension and correct potassium levels before surgery.

18. F ★★★   OH Clin Surg, 4th edn → p257

High dose T_4 replacement is usually indicated in patients who have undergone a total thyroidectomy for thyroid cancer. It is used to suppress the secretion of TSH as evidence suggests that it reduces the risk of local and regional recurrence.

19. I ★   OH Clin Surg, 4th edn → p253

The diagnosis in this case is hyperthyroidism. The first line of treatment in this case is a beta blocker (propranolol) that is used to control both the tremor and tachycardia.

20. E ★★   OH Clin Surg, 4th edn → p256

The most appropriate replacement hormone in this case is T_3 due to its short half life. This can be stopped prior to ^{131}I-whole body scan to allow a rise in TSH and increase the uptake of ^{131}I in any remaining thyroid cells.

Chapter 6

Upper gastrointestinal surgery

James Wood

Diseases of the upper gastrointestinal tract (GI) have changed a great deal both in their aetiology and presentations as well as their management in the last three decades. Modern students and junior doctors need to understand the range of upper GI conditions which now present, especially the increasing issues of upper GI malignancy and the impact of morbid obesity on medical and surgical practice. Old text books full of operations for benign peptic ulcer disease have been replaced with texts on the constantly advancing treatment of oesophagogastric cancer and operations for obesity management.

Symptoms and signs in upper GI disease are often subtle and non-specific so a sound knowledge of clinical findings and the choices for appropriate investigations are extremely important and are covered in this chapter.

Lastly, some of the most urgent and life-threatening surgical emergencies can occur due to upper GI disease and the management of these conditions is a vital area of knowledge for all junior doctors.

Neil Borley

QUESTIONS

Single Best Answers

1. A 28-year-old woman has dysphagia with low retrosternal 'sticking' and an occasional sensation of choking. A video barium swallow shows this appearance in the oesophagus (see Figure 6.1).

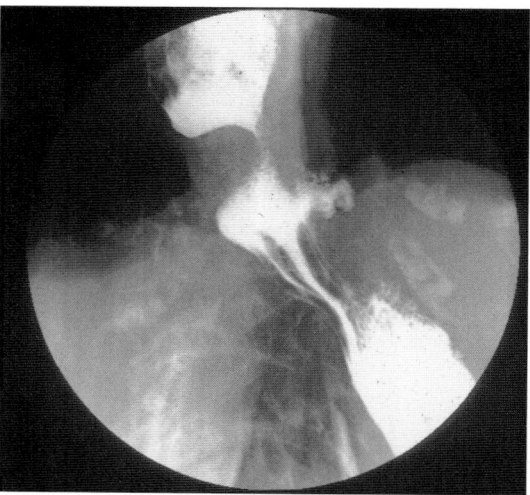

Figure 6.1 Appearance of the oesophagus as shown in the video of the barium swallow

Which is the *single* most likely diagnosis? ★★

A Achalasia

B Carcinoma of the oesophagus

C Diffuse oesophageal spasm

D Foreign body ingestion

E Reflux oesophagitis

2. A junior medical student asks you about the principal differences of macroscopic appearances and functions of the proximal jejunum and distal ileum. Which is the *single* correct statement comparing the features of each? ★

A Compared to the ileum, the jejunum: absorbs less vitamin B_6, is thinner walled, and secretes more fluid during digestion

B Compared to the ileum, the jejunum: absorbs more vitamin B_6, secretes less fluid during digestion, and appears redder in colour

C Compared to the ileum, the jejunum: is thicker walled, possesses less prominent lymphoid tissue, and secretes more fluid during digestion

D Compared to the ileum, the jejunum: possesses less prominent lymphoid tissue, paler and appears blue in colour, absorbs less vitamin B_6

E Compared to the ileum, the jejunum: possesses more prominent lymphoid tissue, appears paler blue in colour, and secretes less fluid during digestion

3. A 72-year-old man has had a sensation of retrosternal burning that is worse at night and after meals for the last 4 months. It partially responds to 'over the counter' antacid treatment. Which is the *single* most appropriate initial diagnostic investigation? ★

A Barium meal

B Barium swallow

C CT scan thorax

D OGD

E 24h pH studies

4. A 64-year-old woman undergoes an oesophagogastroduodenoscopy (OGD) to investigate difficulties and discomfort with swallowing. A tumour is found in the distal oesophagus. Biopsies are taken. Which is the *single* most likely histological diagnosis? ★

A Adenocarcinoma

B GI stromal tumour

C Lipoma

D Rhabdomyosarcoma

E Squamous cell carcinoma

5. A 50-year-old man has a 15-pack-year history of smoking and undergoes an OGD. There is a duodenal ulcer present. Gastric biopsies are taken and undergo a rapid urease test. Which *single* organism is most likely to be identified? ★

A *Clostridium difficile*

B *Escherichia coli*

C *Enterobacter*

D *Helicobacter pylori*

E *Staphylococcus aureus*

6. A 79-year-old man has an incidental finding of a haemoglobin of 9.1g/dL and mean corpuscular volume of 72fL with mild postprandial epigastric pain. Which is the *single* most appropriate first-line investigation? ★

A Barium meal

B CT scan thorax

C MRI upper abdomen

D OGD

E Ultrasound scan upper abdomen

7. A 67-year-old man is found to have adenocarcinoma of the stomach. Which *single* blood group is this pathology associated with? ★

A A

B AB

C B

D O

E None of these

8. A 69-year-old woman with rheumatoid arthritis has had 24h of epigastric pain, abdominal tenderness, and fever. She takes regular ibuprofen and has recently been taking oral steroids. An erect chest X-ray is taken in the emergency department (see Figure 6.2).

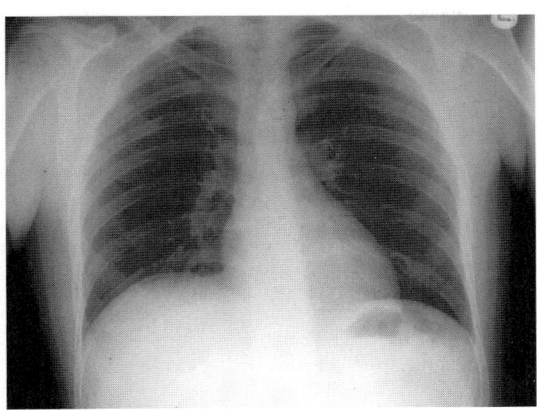

Figure 6.2 An erect chest X-ray is taken

Which is the *single* most likely diagnosis? ★

A Acute pancreatitis

B Bleeding duodenal ulcer

C Incarcerated hiatus hernia

D Perforated peptic ulcer

E Right lower lobe pneumonia

9. A 79-year-old man has been having frequent dark black/bloody semi-liquid and foul smelling stools over the last 24h associated with vague generalized abdominal pain and bloating. His haemoglobin is 12.5g/dL, white blood cell count 11×10^9/L, and serum urea 18mmol/L. Which is the *single* most likely diagnosis? ★

A Angiodysplasia of the stomach

B Bleeding duodenal ulcer

C *Clostridium difficile* colitis

D Colonic carcinoma

E Gastroenteritis

10. An 83-year-old man is admitted with acute onset of severe epigastric pain and has 'board-like' rigidity of the upper abdomen. His temperature is 37.4°C, pulse rate 124bpm, blood pressure 104/75mmHg. A working diagnosis of visceral perforation is made and investigations planned. Which is the *single* most appropriate fluid prescription to administer? ★★

A IV Hartmann's solution 500mL, over 2h

B IV O-negative blood 2 units, run in

C IV sodium bicarbonate 0.13% 500mL, over 2h

D IV sodium chloride 0.9% 100mL, over 2h

E IV whole cross-matched blood 2 units, over 4h

11. A 13-year-old adolescent girl has had 2 days of increasing right iliac fossa and lower abdominal pain with tenderness and guarding. Her temperature is 37.8°C, pulse is 92bpm. A provisional diagnosis of acute appendicitis is made and a laparoscopic appendicectomy planned. Which is the *single* most appropriate investigation prior to the procedure? ★

A Abdominal X-ray

B Chest X-ray

C CT scan abdomen and pelvis

D Pregnancy test

E Transabdominal pelvic ultrasound scan

12. A 6-week-old boy is brought to hospital with projectile and persistent vomiting. Weight gain has been poor. The child appears listless and quiet. A lump is palpable in the upper abdomen. Pulse is 100bpm, serum electrolytes are sodium 132mmol/L and potassium 3.2mmol/L. A provisional diagnosis of pyloric stenosis is made. Which is the *single* most appropriate initial intervention? ★★★

A Administration of IV bicarbonate 8.4% solution (weight adjusted)

B Administration of IV 0.9% sodium chloride (weight adjusted)

C Administration of a test feed

D Commencing nil by mouth

E Insertion of a nasogastric tube

13. An 8-month-old boy is described by his mother as having 3 days of intermittent severe distress and restlessness and the recent passage of bloody motions and mucus-like material. There has been some vomiting and the abdomen is mildly distended and tender to examination. Which is the *single* most likely diagnosis? ★★★

A Gastroenteritis

B Hirschsprung's disease

C Intussusception (ileocaecal)

D Pyloric stenosis

E Small bowel volvulus

14. A 27-year-old woman has had 4 days of gradually increasing, diffuse lower abdominal pain and 6h of acute severe worsening of the pain. Her abdomen is tender with guarding in the lower half. Her temperate is 37.2°C, pulse 104bpm, blood pressure 104/56mmHg, and capillary refill approximately 6sec. Which is the *single* most likely diagnosis? ★★

A Acute tubo-ovarian abscess

B Endometriosis

C Perforated diverticulitis

D Ruptured ectopic pregnancy

E Torted ovarian cyst

Extended Matching Questions

Gastrointestinal investigations

For each scenario choose the *single* most appropriate investigation from the list of options. Each option may be used once, more than once, or not at all.

A Abdominal ultrasound scan

B Barium enema (double contrast)

C Capsular endoscopy

D Colonoscopy

E CT colonography ('CT colonoscopy')

F CT scan of the abdomen

G Endoscopic ultrasound scan

H OGD with duodenal biopsy

I OGD with gastric biopsy

J OGD with oesophageal biopsy

K Small bowel follow through

1. A 34-year-old woman has abdominal discomfort and loose stools after food with a weight loss of 5kg over 12 months and has developed poor skin and hair texture. She has haemoglobin of 8.3g/dL and ferritin of 7mg/dL. ★★

2. A 63-year-old man is under surveillance for Barrett's metaplasia. ★★★

3. A 24-year-old man has had progressive, intermittent right iliac fossa pain with variable loose stools and weight loss of 10kg for 2 years. ★★★

4. An 84-year-old woman with severe chronic obstructive pulmonary disease and chronic renal impairment on long-term oral steroids. She has a palpable right iliac fossa mass. Her haemoglobin is 7.7g/dL and ferritin 9 mg/dL. ★★★

5. A 63-year-old man admitted with upper abdominal pain and melaena for 24h. His heart rate is 108bpm and blood pressure is 98/45mmHg. ★

Gastrointestinal anatomy

For each scenario choose the *single* most appropriate anatomical location for the likely diagnosis from the list of options. Each option may be used once, more than once, or not at all. Figure 6.3 displays the options.

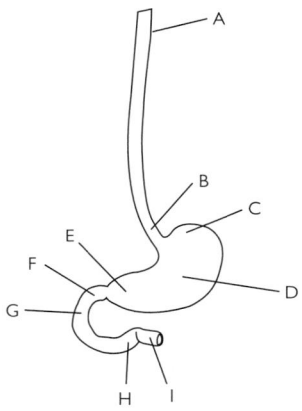

Figure 6.3 Upper gastrointestinal anatomy

6. A 68-year-old man with a 25-pack-year history of smoking takes regular ibuprofen for headaches but denies drinking alcohol. He has had 2 weeks of constant, worsening epigastric pain radiating to the middle of his back and has 6h of passing dark red and black stools with 2h of vomiting clotted red blood. ★★★

7. A 24-year-old woman has several years of worsening difficult, painful swallowing which is worse with fluids than solids, and has recently developed nocturnal coughing and wheezing. ★★★

8. A 53-year-old man undergoes an OGD to investigate dyspepsia. *Helicobacter pylori* is suspected as the cause and biopsies are taken from this location to assess for the presence of the organism. ★

9. A 28-year-old man has abdominal discomfort, weight loss, and diarrhoea. A serum tissue transglutaminase test is positive. An OGD is performed to establish a diagnosis and multiple biopsies are taken from this site. ★★★

10. A 45-year-old man has been vomiting violently for 3h after a take-away meal and the last three episodes of vomiting have been accompanied by streaks of fresh red blood in the vomitus. ★★

Operations for gastrointestinal complaints

For each scenario choose the *single* most appropriate operation from the list of options. Each option may be used once, more than once, or not at all.

A Anti-reflux fundoplication

B Cardiomyotomy ('Heller's operation')

C Duodenotomy and repair

D Gastrojejunal bypass

E Hepaticojejunostomy

F Oesophagectomy

G Pancreaticoduodenectomy

H Partial gastrectomy

I Total gastrectomy

11. A 27-year-old woman has had several years of progressive dysphagia and a 'bird's beak' appearance on barium swallow. Balloon dilatation has failed and she requires surgery. ★★★★

12. A 47-year-old man has a longstanding proven gastro-oesophageal reflux disease and has severe persistent and debilitating symptoms despite maximal medical therapy. ★★★

13. A 52-year-old man has ongoing melaena in hospital. He has a proven proximal duodenal ulcer and has continued bleeding despite two episodes of endoscopic treatment. ★

14. A 67-year-old man with no other medical co-morbidity has a carcinoma of the body of the stomach staged as T2 N0. ★★★

15. A 74-year-old man with invasive adenocarcinoma of the head of the pancreas involving the superior mesenteric vessels. ★★

Gastrointestinal symptoms

For each scenario choose the *single* most likely diagnosis from the list of options. Each option may be used once, more than once, or not at all.

A Adenocarcinoma

B Chronic intestinal ischaemia

C Diffuse oesophageal spasm

D Gastro-oesophageal reflux disease

E Laceration (traumatic)

F Myocardial infarction

G Neuroendocrine tumour ('carcinoid type')

H Peptic ulcer

I Pharyngeal pouch

16. A 25-year-old man undergoes an operation for suspected appendicitis. However, an inflamed Meckel's diverticulum is found and excised. Histopathological examination identifies another pathology within the diverticulum in addition to the inflammation. ★★★★

17. A 22-year-old man with small volume haematemesis following a prolonged episode of vomiting during an evening of binge drinking. ★★★

18. A 76-year-old man with a history of smoking has a 2h history of acute onset epigastric and chest pain. His abdomen is non-tender and his pulse rate is 100bpm. ★

19. A 74-year-old man with months of progressive dysphagia, weight loss of 4kg, and anorexia. ★

20. A 38-year-old man who smokes ten cigarettes/day has retrosternal burning pain after meals especially when lying down. He has some pain on swallowing with a sensation of food becoming 'stuck' in his throat. ★★★

Acute abdominal pain

For each patient with acute abdominal pain choose the *single* most likely diagnosis from the list of options. Each option may be used once, more than once, or not at all.

A Abdominal aortic aneurysm (leaking)

B Acute appendicitis

C Acute cholecystitis

D Acute mesenteric ischaemia

E Acute pancreatitis

F Acute sigmoid diverticulitis

G Acute urinary retention

H Biliary colic

I Renal colic

21. A 52-year-old woman with 48h of epigastric and right-sided abdominal pain, no jaundice, a temperature of 37.8°C, a pulse of 100bpm, and a white blood cell count of 14.7×10^9/L. ★★

22. A 72-year-old man with 2h of severe central and left-sided abdominal pain radiating to the left flank and back. He is feeling faint. He has generalized mild abdominal tenderness but no palpable masses. His pulse rate is 92bpm, blood pressure is 116/80mmHg. ★★★

23. A 47-year-old woman with 3 days of increasing left lower abdominal pain, mild dysuria, and left iliac fossa and left flank tenderness. Her temperature is 37.7°C, pulse is 82bpm, and blood pressure is 135/76 mmHg. The urine is positive for blood and protein and negative for nitrites. ★★★

24. A 52-year-old man with 12h of intermittent colicky right-sided abdominal pain, nausea, and retching. His temperature is 37.4°C, pulse is 82bpm, and blood pressure is 135/85mmHg. ★★

25. An 81-year-old man with some cognitive impairment is reported by his carers to have seemed to have 6h of progressively increasing lower abdominal, left iliac fossa, and suprapubic pain. There is mild lower abdominal tenderness but no obvious mass. His temperature is 37.2°C, pulse is 88bpm, and blood pressure is 155/85mmHg. ★★★

ANSWERS

Single Best Answers

1. A ★★   OH Clin Surg, 4th edn → p274

Achalasia (failure of relaxation of the distal oesophageal musculature associated with degeneration of the myenteric plexus) is among the most common causes of dysphagia in the younger population. This radiological appearance is characteristic of achalasia with a single, smooth, distal oesophageal abnormality where the lumen tapers sharply to a fine point ('bird beak appearance'). The lack of mucosal irregularity makes a tumour very unlikely and diffuse spasm gives a variable multiple level abnormality. A reflux stricture would be very rare at her age and would normally be preceded by a long history of reflux symptoms rather than just dysphagia.

2. C ★   OH Clin Surg, 4th edn → p289

The jejunum is generally thick walled, darker red/more purple in colour, with prominent plicae circulares being a predominantly digestive organ producing the majority of the digestive fluid from the small bowel and performing the majority of the absorption for both main nutritional elements and micronutrients.

The ileum tends to be paler and bluer, thinner walled, with thinner plicae circulares but prominent lymphoid follicles. The only vitamin absorbed predominantly in the distal ileum is B_{12}. Practically, injuries to or loss of the jejunum results in relatively more loss of digestive and absorptive capacity than of the distal ileum but loss of the distal ileum leaves the jejunum which is a mainly secretory organ meaning that fluid loss is likely to be more of a problem.

3. D ★   OH Clin Surg, 4th edn → p280

This man most likely has gastro-oesophageal reflux disease. The differential diagnosis includes oesophageal or gastric malignancy, functional disease, and peptic ulcer disease and the first investigation should be direct visualization of the oesophagus and stomach. A barium swallow would exclude tumours or stricturing but would not assess the mucosal integrity so well or allow biopsies to be taken. Twenty-four-hour pH studies may be useful to evaluate the severity or timing of gastro-oesophageal reflux disease but are not useful for diagnosis.

4. A ★   OH Clin Surg, 4th edn → p282

Adenocarcinoma is by far the commonest malignancy of the oesophagus and typically occurs in the lower half, although it is now the most common diagnosis for a malignant tumour below the cricopharyngeus muscle having exceeded squamous carcinoma in incidence. Lipomas rarely occur in the oesophagus since there is little submucosal tissue (unlike the small bowel and colon where they are not uncommon). Similarly, the amount and distribution of autonomic nervous tissue means that GI stromal tumours are much more common in the stomach than the oesophagus. The oesophagus is the commonest location in the GI tract for rhabdomyosarcoma but it is still a very rare tumour overall.

5. D ★   OH Clin Surg, 4th edn → p284

Duodenal ulceration is frequently associated with *Helicobacter pylori*. The causation is due to increased acid production from the antrum of the stomach, possibly due to loss of suppression in the gastric crypts due to penetration of the gastric mucus layer by certain strains of the organism which results in chronic mucosal gastritis. The presence of the organism can be identified in gastric biopsies with a rapid urease test which is more sensitive than microscopic examination of the biopsies for the presence of the organisms.

Clostridium difficile can be found in the stomach and is not always pathological but when so causes diarrhoea rather than duodenal ulceration.

6. D ★   OH Clin Surg, 4th edn → pp188–9

Although there is no ferritin given, the microcytic nature of the anaemia suggests an iron deficiency most likely due to occult blood loss. In a man of his age, the most likely sites for pathology which might cause this are: the proximal colon, the stomach, the duodenum, and the kidney. The usual investigation strategy is for combined (sequential) OGD and colonoscopy with an abdominopelvic CT scan if these first-line investigations are negative.

7. A ★   OH Clin Surg, 4th edn → p286

Gastric adenocarcinoma is associated with blood group A. Other risk factors include a high smoking exposure history, a diet rich in nitrosamines (e.g. raw fish consumption), and chronic atrophic gastritis.

8. D ★   OH Clin Surg, 4th edn → p284

There is a thin sliver of free gas under the right hemidiaphragm over the liver. This is too small to be a bowel loop and there are no features of change in the lung parenchyma making a linear collapse due to chest infection unlikely. The chest X-ray features are of a perforated viscus. With epigastric pain and a history of taking steroids and NSAIDs the most likely cause is a perforated peptic ulcer.

Acute pancreatitis may give rise to all of the same clinical features but in the absence of extreme complications, visceral perforation is very unlikely. Bleeding duodenal ulcer is also a well-recognized complication of NSAID and steroid medication but a history of bleeding and a degree of haemodynamic instability would be expected. Right lower lobe pneumonia is a notorious mimic of intra-abdominal pathology with symptoms and signs which can be exclusively abdominal at presentation. There is no evidence of radiological features of lower lobe change but that does not exclude the condition, however, the presence of the free gas makes the diagnosis.

9. B ★   OH Clin Surg, 4th edn → p284

The history is of melaena rather than dark colonic bleeding and the raised urea suggests that there has been absorption of protein (in the form of haemoglobin) from the small intestine meaning that the bleeding is likely to be from the duodenum or above. Gastroenteritis rarely causes frank bleeding and a duodenal peptic ulcer is much more common than gastric angiodysplasia.

10. A ★★   OH Clin Surg, 4th edn → p296

This is a classic presentation and the tachycardia and hypotension are usually due to autonomic instability rather than absolute hypovolaemia. The priority is to re-establish the circulating volume rapidly and this is best done with a bolus of isotonic solution. Bleeding is rarely associated with a visceral perforation and thus blood of either type is not indicated. It is also slow to administer making it inappropriate as a direct volume restorative. Neither the bicarbonate nor the 0.18% saline are isotonic thus Hartmann's solution or 0.9% saline would be appropriate. In fact, the exact fluid administered is less important than the rate so the 100mL of saline is inadequate.

11. D ★   OH Clin Surg, 4th edn → p288

The diagnosis of acute appendicitis has been made clinically. Chest X-ray, abdominal X-ray, and pelvic ultrasound cannot reliably make or exclude the diagnosis and will not alter the decision to proceed. CT scanning is contraindicated because of her age. Ovarian disease is unlikely and would best be identified on a transvaginal ultrasound scan which is probably not indicated in a girl of this age. Once the diagnosis has been made, diagnostic laparoscopy with a view to appendicectomy is the procedure of choice. The only diagnosis which would affect this decision is the establishment of pregnancy; thus a pregnancy test is mandatory before proceeding with surgery even at this relatively young age.

12. B ★★★   OH Clin Surg, 4th edn → p430

Hypertrophy of the pylorus can cause a gastric outlet obstruction leading to persistent projectile vomiting. This usually becomes apparent in the first 2 months of life. The vomit is high in potassium and chloride and the child may develop hypochloraemic alkalosis. A nasogastric tube will be very difficult to insert and will do nothing to correct any underlying electrolyte imbalances, neither will making the child nil by mouth. A test feed is helpful for diagnosis but the diagnosis may be assumed and restoration of potential physiological upset is a priority. The most likely problem is alkalosis so bicarbonate is contraindicated particularly in hypertonic concentrations of 8.4%. Isotonic (0.9%) saline is appropriate as a first step since, with provision of sodium and potassium ions, renal function will usually correct the acid–base imbalances automatically.

13. C ★★★   OH Clin Surg, 4th edn → p434

Vomiting, infantile distress, and abdominal bloating are non-specific features which may apply to most of these diagnoses. The age of 8 months is too late for a likely presentation of Hirschsprung's disease and the abnormal stools are not typical at all of pyloric stenosis. Gastroenteritis may produce bloody diarrhoea in severe cases but the episodic nature of the symptoms suggests intestinal colic which is most likely from an obstructive process. Small bowel volvulus will not cause bloody stools thus intussusception is most likely. It typically occurs between the ages of 3 and 10 months. Pain, features of bowel obstruction, and the passage of 'redcurrant jelly' stool are typical.

14. D ★★   OH Clin Surg, 4th edn → p306

The clinical findings clearly indicate that the patient shows signs of hypovolaemic shock which is inconsistent with a torted cyst or endometriosis. This is most likely to be due to blood loss or acute severe sepsis. Both tubo-ovarian abscess and diverticulitis may rupture acutely with a rapid deterioration but the diffuse nature of symptoms and the delayed capillary refill are most consistent with blood loss rather than sepsis making ruptured ectopic pregnancy the most likely cause.

Extended Matching Questions

1. H ★★

This woman has iron deficiency anaemia and the discomfort after eating suggests coeliac disease. Established coeliac disease gives rise to malabsorption of both key nutrients (as suggested by the weight loss) and micronutrients (as suggested by the hair and skin changes). Whilst serum tissue transglutaminase testing is routine, biopsies from the distal duodenum are required to confirm the diagnosis of coeliac disease (villous atrophy with intra-epithelial lymphocytes).

2. J ★★★   OH Clin Surg, 4th edn → p280

Barrett's metaplasia affects the lower part of the oesophagus and is the transformation of squamous to glandular columnar epithelium in the anatomical oesophagus. Surveillance for dysplastic changes involves biopsies from this region to detect potentially premalignant changes of high-grade dysplasia.

3. D ★★★

This man has features of Crohn's disease of the terminal ileum. A small bowel follow through might give information about the terminal ileum but it is not usually diagnostic and is best reserved for assessment of complications of an established diagnosis especially of more proximal disease. Similarly, capsule endoscopy is usually used for diagnosis where CT and colonoscopy have not provided clear evidence. Colonoscopy with terminal ileal intubation is the first-line investigation to attempt to achieve a biopsy proven diagnosis.

4. E ★★★

Iron deficiency anaemia is usually investigated with an OGD and colonoscopy. In this woman, the right iliac fossa findings strongly suggest a colonic neoplasm but colonoscopy is relatively contraindicated by her severe chronic obstructive pulmonary disease and renal impairment. Double-contrast barium enema would assess the right colon and a plain abdominal CT scan would give some information about a right iliac fossa mass but the combination of CT scanning with colonic imaging by preparation and air colonography (sometimes called CT colonoscopy) is more accurate in assessing the right iliac fossa/possible caecal pathology and gives the same staging information as plain abdominal CT scanning.

5. I ★

This man is likely to have an upper GI bleed with a peptic ulcer, gastritis, or undiagnosed varices among the most likely diagnoses. An OGD is required to make the diagnosis and haemostatic therapy may be used to stop the bleeding. Biopsies of oesophageal disease or an active duodenal ulcer are usually contraindicated in acute bleeding. Gastric biopsies may be of use if a gastric carcinoma is suspected.

6. F ★★★   OH Clin Surg, 4th edn → pp284, 294

This patient has a severe upper GI bleed. In the absence of any alcohol history the diagnosis is most likely to be bleeding peptic ulcer. Although gastric ulcers (either in the body or the antrum) may bleed very profusely as here, the lack of haematemesis and the back pain suggest the other likely cause of acute severe upper GI haemorrhage which is a duodenal ulcer with bleeding from the gastroduodenal artery. This is located deep to the posterior wall of the first part of the duodenum.

7. B ★★★   OH Clin Surg, 4th edn → p274

The patient has dysphagia. The progressive nature, her age, and the fact that fluids are more troublesome than solids point to a diagnosis of achalasia. This is characterized by failure of relaxation of the distal oesophagus.

8. E ★

OH Clin Surg, 4th edn → p284

Helicobacter pylori are most commonly found beneath the mucus layer in the pre-pyloric antrum of the stomach. A rapid urease test may be done on biopsies from this area although it is *not* the most accurate test for the presence of the organism; serum antibody status gives information on previous or current exposure but a CO_2 breath test is most sensitive for the active presence of the condition.

9. G ★★★

The diagnosis is coeliac disease; the clinical picture is typical and the tissue transglutaminase is very strongly suggestive of the diagnosis. Biopsies from the duodenum are required to confirm the presence of villous atrophy, crypt hyperplasia, and intra-epithelial (T) lymphocytes. These should be multiple and taken from as far distal in the second part of the duodenum as possible since the first part often fails to demonstrate clear evidence of the disease. It is not usually possible to reach the fourth part of the duodenum (site H) during normal OGD.

10. B ★★

OH Clin Surg, 4th edn → p294

The presentation is typical for a Mallory–Weiss tear of the upper GI tract lining. Although it may occur in the fundus of the stomach, the mucosa is more robust here and the most likely location is the distal oesophagus at the gastro-oesophageal junction.

11. B ★★★★

OH Clin Surg, 4th edn → p274

The diagnosis is achalasia—the sex, age, and presentation are typical. Balloon dilatation can be used in other situations but it is most commonly used in achalasia. Heller's cardiomyotomy is performed (usually laparoscopically) to divide the distal oesophageal muscle fibres to reduce the spasm and relieve the dysphagia.

12. A ★★★

OH Clin Surg, 4th edn → p280

Surgical intervention is indicated in patients with severe resistant symptoms or those with complications despite treatment. The procedure of choice is an anti-reflux procedure designed to increase the dynamic tone around the lower oesophagus and gastro-oesophageal junction. Various procedures to wrap the proximal stomach around the gastro-oesophageal junction have been described but the commonest of these is the Nissen fundoplication.

13. C ★

OH Clin Surg, 4th edn → p294

Bleeding from the posterior part of the proximal duodenum is a common site for upper GI bleeding. Ulcers here are almost always benign but may be life threatening and recurrent bleeding despite endoscopic therapy requires emergency surgery. Occasionally the duodenum is severely damaged and cannot be repaired necessitating a partial gastrectomy but much more commonly duodenotomy and under-running of the bleeding vessel with a suture will control the bleeding vessel.

14. I ★★★ OH Clin Surg, 4th edn → p286

Gastric carcinoma is potentially curable by radical resection provided there is no evidence of metastatic disease. This includes anything more than local lymph node disease. With a staging of T2 the primary is confined to the stomach and N0 indicates no known nodal disease. Thus palliation, such as bypass, is only indicated for those not fit for resection. Being in the body of the stomach it is most likely that radical total gastrectomy is required rather than partial gastrectomy.

15. D ★★ OH Clin Surg, 4th edn → p326

Carcinoma of the pancreas may be amenable to curative surgery depending on location and involvement of local structures. Tumours of the head may be resectable by pancreaticoduodenectomy but involvement of the major vessels effectively renders the tumour incurable. Since the tumour is involving the head, the most likely complication is gastric outlet or duodenal obstruction and a gastrojejunal bypass may be necessary to treat it. Obstruction of the common bile duct may occur but bypasses such as hepaticojejunostomy are rarely necessary with endoscopic and radiological stenting techniques.

16. G ★★★★ OH Clin Surg, 4th edn → p292

Meckel's diverticula can be associated with 'peptic' ulceration due to the presence of gastric acid-secreting mucosa but the perforation occurs in the normal ileal wall adjacent to the diverticulum. The small bowel is the commonest site of neuroendocrine tumours, the most common of which is a carcinoid tumour and aberrant tissue, such as a Meckel's diverticulum, may show a predilection for such tumours.

17. E ★★★ OH Clin Surg, 4th edn → p294

Violent vomiting can cause a traumatic laceration in the lining of the oesophagus leading to bleeding and haematemesis (Mallory–Weiss tear). Peptic ulcer disease is possible but the history of preceding vomiting is typical and the shortness of history is again peptic ulcer disease.

18. F ★ OH Clin Surg, 4th edn → p302

Surgeons must be aware of medical conditions that can mimic surgical pathology. Epigastric and chest pain may be due to peptic ulcer disease or intestinal ischaemia but the shortness of the history and the absence of abdominal signs make these less likely and ischaemic heart disease more so. All such patients should have an ECG and the interpretation should be documented in the medical notes.

19. A ★   OH Clin Surg, 4th edn ➜ pp282, 288

Weight loss and anorexia may be features of chronic intestinal ischaemia or peptic ulcer disease but the presence of dysphagia makes a tumour of the oesophagus most likely. Carcinoid tumours are very rarely a cause for the symptoms and adenocarcinoma is the most likely diagnosis.

20. D ★★★   OH Clin Surg, 4th edn ➜ p280

Adenocarcinoma of oesophagus, gastro-oesophageal reflux disease, diffuse spasm, and a pharyngeal pouch may all present with problems with swallowing. The burning pain and pain on lying are much more suggestive of the presence of reflux. Spasm may be extremely difficult to differentiate from gastro-oesophageal reflux disease and may present many similar symptoms but simply on the basis of frequency, gastro-oesophageal reflux disease is the more likely diagnosis.

21. C ★★   OH Clin Surg, 4th edn ➜ p302

The pain is associated with clear features of an inflammatory origin so simple biliary colic, renal colic (without superadded infection), and leaking abdominal aortic aneurysm are all less likely. The origin in the epigastrium makes appendicitis less likely and the presence of pain on the right makes pancreatitis similarly less likely leaving acute cholecystitis as the most likely cause. The absence of jaundice simply means there is no cholangitis or secondary bile duct swelling or compression (Mirizzi syndrome).

22. A ★★★   OH Clin Surg, 4th edn ➜ p302

The combination of short-lived severe pain and haemodynamic upset (he is almost certainly hypotensive for his age and mildly tachycardic) suggests a non-inflammatory cause. Biliary or renal colic may be severe but the relative hypotension is uncharacteristic. Acute mesenteric ischaemia typically causes severe pain but often gives rise to no abdominal signs. The lack of a palpable, pulsatile mass should never be taken as evidence against an abdominal aortic aneurysm and the age and gender of the patient are typical of the diagnosis.

23. F ★★★   OH Clin Surg, 4th edn ➜ p302

The differential lies between left renal colic, sigmoid diverticulitis, and urinary tract infection. The duration and onset all point strongly to diverticulitis. The presence of blood and protein in the urine without the presence of nitrites is against urinary infection and can be explained by inflammation of the dome of the bladder by an adjacent loop of inflamed sigmoid colon.

24. H ★★   OH Clin Surg, 4th edn → p302

The short history and colicky nature of the pain makes an inflammatory process such as acute appendicitis less likely although still possible. The nausea and retching favour a biliary or upper GI origin to the pain rather than renal colic and although there is a mild tachycardia, this is most likely to be due to pain rather than inflammation making biliary colic the most likely diagnosis.

25. G ★★★   OH Clin Surg, 4th edn → p302

Lower abdominal pain can be difficult to differentiate, especially in the elderly. The absence of fever is against the presence of an infective or inflammatory cause but one should be cautious in the elderly as the temperature may be 'falsely' kept low. The mild hypertension may be normal for him but is typical of distress related to autonomic-derived pain as is the tachycardia. A diagnosis of sigmoid diverticulitis must be considered but a trial catheterization should be undertaken first even if the bladder is not obviously distended as urinary retention is a common cause for these symptoms in this age and cognitive state.

Chapter 7

Hepatobiliary surgery

James Wood

The reaction of most students to questions about hepatobiliary disease is a sinking feeling of despair! 'Lots of biochemistry and anatomy together with a bunch of funny eponymous syndromes to remember!' Well, hepatobiliary disease is remarkably logical; knowledge of the basic principles of biliary metabolism and the key anatomical facts is usually more than enough if it is coupled with a sound appreciation of the common clinical presentations.

These presentations are extremely common; most days on call will see the surgical team looking after at least one patient with one of the range of hepatopancreaticobiliary problems that can present as an emergency.

This chapter will review the basic principles of liver and pancreatic disease and the anatomy that goes with it. Both elective and emergency surgical presentations will also be covered, allowing you to revise knowledge of key clinical presentations in practice.

Neil Borley

QUESTIONS

Single Best Answers

1. A 42-year-old woman attends the emergency department with severe epigastric pain after eating fish and chips. The pain resolves after 2h. Her temperature is 37.2°C. She has no abdominal tenderness and all blood investigations are within the normal range. Which is the *single* most likely diagnosis? ★

A Biliary colic

B Cholangitis

C Cholecystitis

D Pancreatitis

E Perforated gallbladder

2. A 48-year-old woman has had progressively worsening colicky abdominal pain for 48h which has become severe and constant for the last 12h. There is a past history of an abdominal hysterectomy. The abdomen is slightly distended but non-tender. Blood investigations are normal except for a white cell count of 13×10^9/L. Which is the *single* most likely diagnosis? ★★

A Acute cholecystitis

B Acute pancreatitis

C Ascending cholangitis

D Ischaemic bowel

E Perforated peptic ulcer

3. A 48-year-old man has been vomiting fresh blood with clots for 3h. He drinks 40 units of alcohol per week. A gastroscopy is performed within 12h and reveals evidence of bleeding from oesophageal varices. Which is the *single* most likely cause of his varices? ★★

A Alcoholic gastritis

B Budd–Chiari syndrome (hepatic vein thrombosis)

C Essential hypertension

D Pancreatitis

E Portal hypertension

4. A 47-year-old woman has 12h of progressive onset epigastric and upper abdominal pain and rigors with temperatures up to 39.2°C. Her pulse is 102bpm, blood pressure is 110/70mmHg, and there is mild jaundice present. Which is the *single* most likely diagnosis? ★★★

A Ascending cholangitis

B Biliary colic

C Cholecystitis—acute

D Empyema of the gallbladder

E Hepatic failure

5. An 82-year-old man has a diagnosis of inoperable cancer of the head of the pancreas. He has developed jaundice over the last 5 days and is symptomatic with pruritus. An abdominal ultrasound scan confirms dilated common and intrahepatic bile ducts. Which is the *single* most suitable means of palliation for his jaundice? ★★★

A Chlorpheniramine PO

B Choledochojejunostomy

C Endoscopic retrograde cholangiopancreatography (ERCP) and internal stent

D Naloxone IV

E Percutaneous transhepatic external drain

6. A 46-year-old woman has a 24h history of sudden onset of constant epigastric pain radiating to the back with nausea. There is central and upper abdominal tenderness. The amylase is 1642IU. Which is the *single* most likely aetiology for the presenting condition? ★

A Alcohol

B Combined oral contraceptive pill

C Gallstones

D Hyperlipidaemia

E Systemic viral infection

7. A 52-year-old man has been drinking up to 30 units of alcohol per week and has longstanding epigastric pain. He has had multiple admissions to hospital with pain. He is admitted with further epigastric pain, mild epigastric tenderness, a white cell count of 7×10^9/L, and an amylase of 102IU. Which is the *single* most likely diagnosis? ★★

A Acute pancreatitis

B Biliary colic

C Chronic pancreatitis

D Hiatus hernia

E Intestinal ischaemia

8. A 43-year-old man has had multiple previous admissions for alcohol-related problems and has had 2h of acute vomiting with copious amounts of bright and dark red blood. An urgent OGD has shown the cause to be bleeding oesophageal varices which have been banded but the vomiting of blood continues on the ward. An anaesthetist is present who has established IV access and is administering blood and fluid transfusions. Which is the *single* most important next step in this patient's management? ★★★

A Take blood for clotting and LFTs

B Contact endoscopy to arrange a further endoscopy

C Contact X-ray to arrange a portable chest-ray

D Contact X-ray to arrange an emergency CT scan with embolization

E Contact your consultant to discuss transfer to theatre for treatment

9. A 23-year-old woman undergoes a laparoscopic cholecystectomy for symptoms of recurrent biliary colic. On examination of the gallbladder there are stones present (see Figure 7.1).

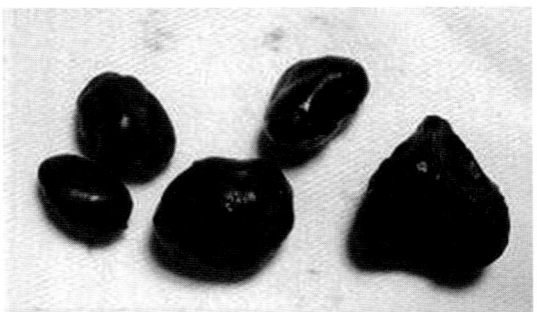

Figure 7.1 Gallbladder stones found on investigation
© Dr Tom Guest

Which is the *single* most likely underlying diagnosis to explain her condition? ★★★★

A Crigler–Najjar syndrome

B Gilbert's syndrome

C Hereditary spherocytosis

D Hypercholesterolaemia

E Pregnancy

10. A 47-year-old man has had malaise and anorexia for 2 weeks and 3 days of developing jaundice. Serum testing has confirmed a positive result for hepatitis A infection. Blood tests are taken to assess the cause of his jaundice (normal values at your hospital are given in Table 7.1).

Table 7.1 Normal blood values

Bilirubin	3–17µmol/L
Alkaline phosphatase (ALP)	30–140IU/L
Alanine aminotransferase (ALT)	3–35IU/L
Aspartate aminotranferase (AST)	3–35IU/L
Creatine kinase (CK)	25–195IU/L
Gamma glutamyl transferase (γGT)	5–50IU/L
Lactate dehydrogenase (LDH)	70–250IU/L

Which is the *single* most likely combination of blood results in this patient? ★★★

A ALP 270IU/L, ALT 27IU/L, AST 37IU/L

B ALP 330IU/L, ALT 105IU/L, CK 350IU/L

C ALP 105IU/L, ALT 75IU/L, AST 60IU/L

D ALP 450IU/L, ALT 55IU/L, γGT 120IU/L

E ALT 130IU/L, AST 25IU/L, LDH 135IU/L

11. A 48-year-old woman has recently undergone extensive bowel resection for complications of ischaemia and has been receiving total parenteral nutrition via a conventional central line. There is currently mild abdominal discomfort and a non-productive cough. There is no evidence of anaemia or jaundice. She has developed a swinging pyrexia as high as 39.5°C over the last 12h. Which is the *single* most likely diagnosis? ★★★

A Acute cholangitis

B Acute respiratory distress syndrome

C Central venous line infection

D Deep vein thrombosis

E Pneumonia

12. A 43-year-old man is referred by his GP with ongoing abdominal pain, vomiting, and a persistent raised temperature several weeks after an episode of acute pancreatitis. There is a palpable upper abdominal mass. Which is the *single* most likely diagnosis? ★★★

A Abdominal aortic aneurysm

B Carcinoma of the pancreas

C Empyema of the gallbladder

D Pseudocyst of the lesser sac

E Small bowel obstruction

13. A 47-year-old woman has had intermittent epigastric discomfort and dyspepsia after food for 10 months. OGD reveals features of moderate inflammation in the body and antrum of the stomach without gastric or duodenal ulceration. A rapid urease test from a biopsy is positive. Which is the *single* most appropriate treatment prescription for her? ★★★

A Gaviscon 10mL PO as needed + omeprazole 20mg once daily

B Omeprazole 20mg PO twice daily + amoxicillin 250mg PO three times daily

C Omeprazole 20mg PO twice daily + metronidazole 400mg PO twice daily + clarithromycin 250mg PO twice daily

D Omeprazole 20mg PO twice daily + ranitidine 150mg PO twice daily

E Ranitidine 150mg PO twice daily + metronidazole 400mg PO twice daily + amoxicillin 250mg PO three times daily

14. A 78-year-old man has acute severe pancreatitis caused by alcohol. His results are shown in Table 7.2.

Table 7.2 Blood results in a patient with acute severe pancreatitis

Serum amylase	1024IU
Serum corrected calcium	2.3mmol/L
White cell count	17×10^9/L
Serum glucose	12mmol/L
Albumin	40g/L
PaO_2	14kPa

Which is his *single* correct Glasgow severity score? ★★

A 1

B 2

C 3

D 4

E 5

15. A 62-year-old man has an adenocarcinoma of the head of the pancreas at the ampulla of Vater. There is no evidence of distant disease and no obvious loco-regional involvement on CT scanning. He is considered for potentially curative treatment. Which is the *single* most appropriate operation for him to be offered? ★★★

A Cholecystectomy

B Distal pancreatectomy

C Gastrojejunostomy

D Pancreaticoduodenectomy

E Radical gastrectomy

Extended Matching Questions

Investigating hepatobiliary complaints

For each scenario choose the *single* most appropriate investigation to achieve the diagnosis from the list of options. Each option may be used once, more than once, or not at all.

A Abdominal X-ray

B Barium meal and follow through

C CT scan of the abdomen

D CT cholangiogram

E Endoscopic retrograde cholangiopancreatography (ERCP)

F Endoscopic ultrasound scan (biliary)

G OGD

H Magnetic resonance cholangiopancreatography (MRCP)

I Upper abdominal ultrasound scan

1. A 37-year-old woman has had 3 days of increasing epigastric pain, nausea, and fever. She is tender in the right upper quadrant of the abdomen. Investigations reveal a WBC of 17×10^9/L, a CRP of 25mg/L, and an aspartate transaminase of 67IU/L. ★

2. A 62-year-old man has had epigastric pain developing jaundice, pale stools, and dark urine for 1 week. An ultrasound scan has shown gallstones in the gallbladder and a common bile duct diameter of 10mm. ★★

3. A 72-year-old woman is seen in clinic following an attack of acute pancreatitis. A recent ultrasound scan has demonstrated gallstones in the gallbladder and a probable stone in the common bile duct. She is being considered for a laparoscopic cholecystectomy. ★★★

4. A 79-year-old man has had intermittent episodes of colicky epigastric pain, abdominal distension, and vomiting for 2 weeks. His abdomen is distended, tympanitic, but there is no evidence of tenderness or peritonism. ★★★

5. A 72-year-old woman has had persistent and increasing epigastric pain with a loss of appetite and some pain after eating for 5 weeks. Abdominal examination is normal. ★★★

Hepatobiliary anatomical structures

For each scenario choose the *single* most appropriate anatomical structure from the list of options. Each option may be used once, more than once, or not at all. Figure 7.2 displays the options.

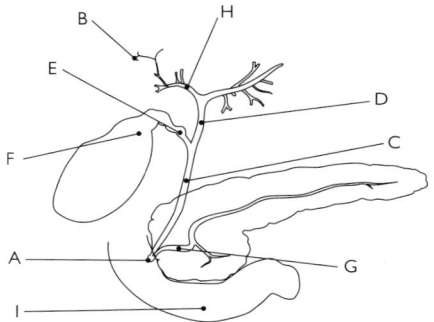

Figure 7.2 Hepatobiliary anatomical structures

6. A 47-year-old woman has recurrent episodes of epigastric pain and right upper quadrant after eating typically lasting 30min to 1h. ★★★

7. During a laparoscopic cholecystectomy the surgeon should identify and divide this structure which forms the inferior side of Calot's triangle. ★★★

8. During an endoscopic retrograde cholangiopancreatography the endoscopist identifies and passes a cannula into this structure to take the required images. ★★★

9. A 48-year-old woman has obstructive jaundice due to Mirizzi's syndrome. There is external compression to this structure. ★★★★

10. A patient admitted to hospital with pancreatitis undergoes an ERCP to remove stones from this structure. ★★

Nutritional delivery methods

For each scenario choose the *single* most appropriate means of nutritional delivery from the list of options. Each option may be used once, more than once, or not at all.

A Any oral fluids and food

B Any oral fluids only

C Clear oral fluids only

D Feeding jejunostomy

E Nasogastric feeding

F Nasojejunal feeding

G Nil feeding

H Percutaneous endoscopic gastrostomy tube

I Total parenteral nutrition

11. A patient is due to undergo an ultrasound scan of the gallbladder in 4h time. ★★

12. A patient is undergoing a major operation involving the stomach, duodenum, and pancreas and they will require postoperative supplemental nutrition. ★★★★

13. A patient with dysphagia and an 'unsafe' swallow reflex following a stroke requires a means of delivering long-term nutrition. ★★

14. A patient is suffering a prolonged ileus due to profound small bowel swelling caused by severe pancreatitis and requires nutrition during a likely prolonged stay in intensive care. ★

15. A patient has just undergone a laparoscopic cholecystectomy. ★★★

Hepatobiliary tumours

For each scenario choose the *single* type of tumour which is most likely to be responsible for the presentation from the list of options. Each option may be used once, more than once, or not at all.

A Adenocarcinoma of pancreas

B Cholangiocarcinoma

C Gastrinoma

D Hepatocellular carcinoma

E Insulinoma

F Liposarcoma

G Mucinous cystadenocarcinoma of pancreas

H Pancreatic blastoma

I VIPoma

16. A 37-year-old man has had 9 months of worsening epigastric pain, weight loss, and loose stools despite acid reduction treatment and at gastroscopy is found to have extensive multifocal ulceration of the stomach and duodenum including the second part. There are no obvious masses associated. ★★★

17. A 76-year-old man has had 4 months of 5kg weight loss and anorexia with 10 days of developing painless jaundice. ★

18. A 32-year-old woman has had 18 months of episodic lethargy, sweating, and episodes of aggressive behaviour often precipitated by hunger and which cease after eating. ★★★★

19. A 35-year-old woman has had 12 months of prolonged watery diarrhoea, lethargy, and dehydration. Serum sodium is 124mmol/L and potassium 3.4mmol/L. ★★★★

20. A 71-year-old man drinks 35 units of alcohol per week, has proven hepatitis C, and has had 2 months of anorexia, anergia, weight loss of 3kg, and epigastric fullness on examination. ★★

ANSWERS

Single Best Answers

1. A ★ — OH Clin Surg, 4th edn → p317

Biliary colic is severe epigastric pain caused by gallstones that typically lasts for half an hour or more and then eases off. Precipitation by foods high in fat is common due to the stimulating effect on cholecystokinin release which increases gallbladder contraction. There may or may not be right subcostal radiation. The absence of signs or features of inflammation or infection make cholecystitis or cholangitis unlikely and the short-lived nature makes pancreatitis very unlikely.

2. D ★★ — OH Clin Surg, 4th edn → p302

The symptoms would be consistent with several diagnoses but the most important feature is the disproportion between the severe symptoms and minimal physical signs. This is always highly suggestive of intestinal ischaemia. An urgent CT scan is the diagnostic test of choice although if the patient is rapidly deteriorating, sometimes emergency surgery is directly indicated.

3. E ★★ — OH Clin Surg, 4th edn → p302

Varices (oesophageal and gastric) are most commonly caused by increased portal venous pressure. This is commonly caused by liver cirrhosis and alcohol-related liver injury is the most common cause in the UK. Increased portal venous pressure causes the development of dilated vessels and increased blood flow through the portosystemic anastomoses particularly around the lower oesophagus and upper stomach. These dilated vessels are prone to incidental trauma and resulting profuse bleeding. Hepatic venous thrombosis causes increased hepatic venous pressure but, unless this is very longstanding with subsequent liver fibrosis and damage, the portal venous pressure is not usually greatly raised.

Gastritis and pancreatitis are associated with alcohol use but not the presence of varices. Systemic arterial (essential) hypertension does not affect portal venous pressure.

4. A ★★★ — OH Clin Surg, 4th edn → p318

This clinical syndrome seen in ascending cholangitis is known as Charcot's triad. The epigastric pain is non-diagnostic but the jaundice is indicative of hepatocellular dysfunction and common bile duct obstruction. The high fever or rigors is specific for common bile duct infection rather than gallbladder sepsis since the organisms more readily enter the bloodstream via the upper biliary tree.

5. C ★★★   OH Clin Surg, 4th edn → p327

This man almost certainly has jaundice due to external compression of the bile duct. Although antihistamines may be helpful acutely to reduce the symptoms of pruritus, the most important thing is to reduce his bilirubin by achieving adequate drainage of the common bile duct and bile flow. Even palliative bypass surgery should be avoided if at all possible; it has a high morbidity and mortality rate in patients with advanced malignancy. A percutaneous external drain is uncomfortable and not a definitive solution other than in terminal care where the life expectancy is very short. It may be used as a prelude to attempting a combined endoscopic and transcutaneous 'rendezvous' procedure. If it can be done a stent placed at ERCP is most likely to be effective in the medium term. Although it may require to be replaced, most stents will allow relief of jaundice for up to 3 months. Naloxone IV in low doses is used to relieve the pruritus of morphine administration which might complicate this man's care but it is not the cause of the symptom here.

6. C ★   OH Clin Surg, 4th edn → p332

This lady has acute pancreatitis. The mnemonic GET SMASHED lists the possible causes (Gallstones, Ethanol, Trauma, Steroids, Mumps (and other viruses), Autoimmune diseases, Hypercalcaemia/Hyperlipidaemia, ERCP, Drugs). As suggested by the list order, the commonest cause in the UK is gallstones with the second commonest being alcohol. Although no history of gallstones is given, at her age this remains the most likely although close review of alcohol intake history, even modest amounts, is necessary and the diagnosis must always be confirmed with abdominal ultrasound scanning, ideally within 24h of admission.

7. C ★★   OH Clin Surg, 4th edn → p320

Chronic epigastric pain accompanied by long-term alcohol excess can lead to chronic pancreatitis. The pain is typically recurrent often with no features of significant inflammation (i.e. normal white cell count and amylase). This may lead to recurrent hospital admissions for pain control. The recurrent nature of the symptoms and the lack of a raised white cell count or amylase is against this being acute pancreatitis and makes intestinal ischaemia very unlikely. Hiatus hernia might give rise to epigastric pain but retrosternal pain and problems with swallowing might be expected. Biliary colic is possible since the associated pain is not always right upper quadrant but it would be less likely in a 52-year-old man with a history of alcohol use.

8. E ★★★   OH Clin Surg, 4th edn → p330

Failed endoscopic therapy with active ongoing bleeding is an indication for emergency 'surgical' control of the bleeding. There are two possible treatments if the patient is considered for active treatment. Emergency radiological portosystemic shunting procedures can be done (transjugular intrahepatic portosystemic shunt) but they are complex and difficult to arrange quickly. In the presence of active bleeding the most likely way of stabilizing the patient is with a Sengstaken–Blakemore tube (oesophagogastric tube with compression balloons and drainage channels to control the bleeding of oesophageal and/or gastric varices by direct compression). The anaesthetic team are best placed to continue the resuscitation and monitoring of the situation including bloods and basic investigations. The patient is too unstable to be transported to X-ray. You are best placed to arrange the transfer to theatre where the tube can be placed. A Sengstaken–Blakemore tube consists of two (or more) inflatable balloons. The tube is inserted via the mouth into the stomach. The gastric balloon is inflated and gentle traction is applied. The oesophageal balloon is then inflated and the combination of pressures occludes the bleeding varices. It is uncomfortable and usually requires general anaesthesia. Once control has been established, other radiological interventions may be appropriate.

9. C ★★★★   OH Clin Surg, 4th edn → p312

All of these conditions may give rise to jaundice. Gilbert's syndrome and Crigler–Najjar syndrome are causes of jaundice but do not give rise to the formation of gallstones being conditions affecting hepatocellular processing of bilirubin. The stones are dark black which means they have a very high proportion of bilirubin present. Pregnancy and hypercholesterolaemia may affect the proportion of cholesterol in the bile but high bilirubin production most commonly comes from increased breakdown of red blood cells. Hereditary spherocytosis leads to red cell membrane abnormalities which reduce the life span of the cells and leads to chronic haemolysis with pigment stones being a common feature. This fits with the young age of the patient.

10. C ★★★   OH Clin Surg, 4th edn → p312

The most likely diagnosis is a viral hepatitis which fits with the clinical picture and the positive hepatitis A result. In viral hepatitis the commonest pattern of enzyme abnormalities is an increase in hepatocellular enzymes (ALT, AST, γGT, and LDH) but no change in membrane enzymes (ALP) unless there is secondary oedema within the liver tissue causing obstructive changes. CK is not a hepatocellular enzyme but is raised in abnormalities of muscles (skeletal or cardiac) (as in B).

It would be extremely unlikely for one hepatocellular enzyme to be raised without the others (as in E).

11. C ★★★

Central venous line sepsis is a common complication of total parenteral nutrition which is usually administered via a central line. It is typified by a high swinging fever with rigors but little else in the way of symptoms. Acute cholangitis may occur in total parenteral nutrition administration where there are long-term abnormalities of bile flow and an increased risk of stasis with infection but the timescale makes this unlikely as does the absence of jaundice. All the other origins of sepsis tend to produce lower, more persistent temperatures. The feed should be stopped. It may be possible to 'clear' the line with antibiotics but it may be necessary to remove it and send the tip for microbiological culture.

12. D ★★★   OH Clin Surg, 4th edn → p333

Pancreatic pseudocysts can form after an attack of acute pancreatitis. They are a collection of fluid formed from a coalescence of pancreatic fluid formed during the acute attack which lies in the lesser sac between stomach and pancreas, usually sterile, enclosed by fibrous or inflammatory tissue. They can cause gastric irritation and nausea/vomiting or occasionally compression of the duodenum but the commonest presentation is persisting pain and an epigastric mass.

Carcinoma of the pancreas is never caused by an acute attack but occasionally may be the precipitating cause. It is unlikely that the mass is palpable now and wasn't at the time of the acute presentation and the symptoms of vomiting and raised temperature make this very unlikely.

Empyema of the gallbladder would tend to be palpable in the right upper quadrant and would be an uncommon coincidence after an episode of pancreatitis.

A leaking abdominal aortic aneurysm would usually present with haemodynamic instability rather than pyrexia and vomiting is a rare association.

13. C ★★★   OH Clin Surg, 4th edn → p284

This patient has gastritis and gaviscon is a reasonable symptomatic treatment and ranitidine is also effective at symptom control but less so at acid suppression. Both could be used for simple gastritis. The positive fast urease result (e.g. Clotest®) indicates that the underlying cause of the gastritis is almost certainly *Helicobacter pylori* and thus first-line treatment should include combination eradication therapy. This requires acid suppression (omeprazole and lansoprazole are used but not ranitidine) as well as antibacterial therapy. Amoxicillin is effective against *Helicobacter pylori* but should not be used alone and the dose is too small (usually 1g PO twice a day).

14. C ★★   OH Clin Surg, 4th edn → p333

Whilst amylase is used to diagnose acute pancreatitis the actual amylase level does not predict severity. In the modified Glasgow severity score a point is given for each of the following:

Age >55 years	(age 78 = +1)
WBC >15 × 10⁹/L	(17 = +1)
Glucose >7mmol/L	(12= +1)
Albumin <35g/L	(40 = 0)
Corrected Ca <2mmol/L	(2.3 = 0)
PaO₂ <10kPa	(14 = 0)

15. D ★★★   OH Clin Surg, 4th edn → p327

Whipple's operation (pancreaticoduodenectomy) is the only potential curative option for carcinoma of the head of the pancreas. It involves *en bloc* resection of the first and second parts of the duodenum, the distal stomach, the head of the pancreas with the distal common bile duct, and the gallbladder. Although cholecystectomy is part of the procedure, it is not a treatment for pancreatic cancer alone. Radical gastrectomy may be used for gastric cancer and distal pancreatectomy for problems of the tail of the pancreas (usually benign). Gastrojejunostomy is a palliative procedure used to treat obstruction of the duodenum caused by advanced pancreatic cancer.

Unfortunately the majority of cases of carcinoma of the pancreas either have distant metastases or involvement of vital structures around the pancreas (e.g. mesenteric vessels) at the time of presentation which preclude curative treatment.

Extended Matching Questions

1. I ★   OH Clin Surg, 4th edn → p316

This woman has symptoms and signs consistent with acute cholecystitis. An ultrasound scan should confirm the diagnosis and assess the status of the gallbladder inflammation. Although a CT scan would also likely give the diagnosis, the ultrasound will give more information about the status of the gallbladder and the common bile duct and CT scanning involves a significant radiation exposure for a woman of childbearing age.

2. H ★★   OH Clin Surg, 4th edn → p313

This man has obstructive jaundice which is likely to be due to an obstructed bile duct since it is distended. The ultrasound scan has not demonstrated a cause. An MRCP is the investigation of choice to assess the extrahepatic bile duct system and will also give information about the pancreatic ducts. It is the investigation of choice since it is non-invasive (as opposed to an ERCP) and avoids radiation exposure (as in a CT cholangiogram).

3. E ★★★   OH Clin Surg, 4th edn → p333

This woman most likely has pancreatitis caused by a common bile duct stone. Some stones will pass spontaneously into the duodenum but for those that don't removal is required. An ERCP offers a combined investigation to confirm the diagnosis and exclude another cause such as a stricture of the bile duct as well as the option to intervene to remove the stone if possible. An MRCP will confirm the diagnosis of a common bile duct stone but will not allow treatment. Surgery can be used to explore the common bile duct and remove stones but it is commonest to attempt to diagnose and remove these prior to surgery.

4. C ★★★

This man has features of possible bowel obstruction. Although an abdominal X-ray may show features of obstruction, a CT scan is more likely to reveal the diagnosis and the possible cause as well as exclude other mimics of the symptoms such as pseudo-obstruction, acute ascites, or an abdominal mass. A barium meal is contraindicated since, if he were to proceed to surgery, the upper GI tract would be full of radio-opaque fluid.

5. G ★★★

This woman's features are strongly suggestive of gastric pathology. The differential diagnosis includes ulceration, gastritis, and malignancy. OGD offers the opportunity to diagnose the problem with the chance of histological confirmation. Although a barium meal may diagnose a malignancy or a large ulcer, gastritis may not be seen and it does not provide histology. A CT scan alone is notoriously poor at assessing the stomach.

6. F ★★★ OH Clin Surg, 4th edn → p316

The history is typical for biliary colic (severe epigastric pain that often lasts 30min or more). There may or may not be radiation under the right subcostal margin. This is typically caused by irritation or transient impaction of gallstones into the neck of the gallbladder or Hartmann's pouch.

7. E ★★★ OH Clin Surg, 4th edn → p317

The cystic duct connects the gallbladder to the biliary tree. It runs from the neck of the gallbladder to the hepatic duct. It must be divided in order to remove the gallbladder.

8. A ★★★ OH Clin Surg, 4th edn → pp272, 333

When the endoscope is in the duodenum the endoscopist must identify the ampulla of Vater which is cannulated with a guidewire to facilitate access into the common bile duct.

9. D ★★★★ OH Clin Surg, 4th edn → pp316, 770

Mirizzi's syndrome is caused by external compression of the common hepatic duct caused by swelling, usually due to chronic inflammation in the gallbladder which affects the extrahepatic bile duct below the hilum of the liver. Occasionally the compression also affects the common bile duct (the part of the extrahepatic biliary tree below the entry of the cystic duct) but this is not usually isolated.

10. C ★★ OH Clin Surg, 4th edn → pp162, 328

Pancreatitis is most commonly caused by gallstones that have passed into the common bile duct. They can be removed at ERCP.

11. C ★★   OH Clin Surg, 4th edn → p66

Anything ingested containing amino acids or complex carbohydrates will lead to release of GI tract hormones which stimulate the gallbladder to contract and thus make views more difficult to obtain and less reliable. Clear fluids do not and so may be taken freely.

12. F ★★★★   OH Clin Surg, 4th edn → p66

Any major operation involving these organs will mean that the conventional oral route for feeding will not be available to the patient for at least several days. Food must be delivered to the jejunum to ensure it does not interfere with the healing of the surgical sites. It is possible to site a feeding jejunostomy at the time of surgery to facilitate postoperative nutrition but a long, fine-bore nasojejunal tube is easier to look after and is associated with fewer complications.

13. H ★★   OH Clin Surg, 4th edn → p66

If a patient has dysphagia and an unsafe swallow after a stroke they are at high risk of aspiration, then an alternative means of delivering nutrition is required. A percutaneous endoscopic gastrostomy tube is inserted with the aid of a gastroscope and can provide nutrition in the long term. A nasogastric tube is not a long-term solution and may provoke gastro-oesophageal reflux which would also risk aspiration.

14. I ★   OH Clin Surg, 4th edn → p66

If the gut is not functioning then parenteral nutrition is required if it is likely that it will be some time before enteral nutrition can be resumed. Nasal or directly administered nutrition will not be adequately absorbed to provide full nutritional requirements in an acutely unwell patient. It may be used in addition to total parenteral nutrition since a small volume of liquid feed in the gut promotes mucosal health and blood flow.

15. A ★★★   OH Clin Surg, 4th edn → p66

After a laparoscopic cholecystectomy normal nutrition can be resumed as soon as the patient feels able although it may be reasonable to limit food intake to small portions initially.

16. C ★★★   OH Clin Surg, 4th edn → p284

A gastrinoma is a tumour of the pancreas. Increased gastrin secretion leads to excess acid production by the stomach that can lead to ulceration which is typically extensive and involves the distal duodenum which is very rarely involved with simple ulcers or those related to *Helicobacter* infection.

17. A ★   OH Clin Surg, 4th edn → p326

Painless jaundice and weight loss in an elderly person is very suspicious for malignancy. Although jaundice is possible with extensive, multifocal hepatocellular carcinoma, a tumour of the head of the pancreas is a much more likely cause of obstructive jaundice without pain.

18. E ★★★★   OH Clin Surg, 4th edn → p767

This is Whipple's triad of fasting hypoglycaemic attacks, relieved by glucose and associated with raised insulin levels. Although inappropriate insulin administration and some rare metabolic disorders can give rise to these features, the only tumour to do so is an insulinoma, usually found in the body or tail of the pancreas.

19. I ★★★★

The features are of a secretory diarrhoea. There are a number of causes but of the tumours listed only those which are hormonally active would give rise to this picture. A VIPoma is a rare endocrine tumour of non-beta-islet cells and the activity of the upper small bowel provoked by the excess VIP causes watery diarrhoea, dehydration, hypokalaemia, and achlorhydria.

20. D ★★   OH Clin Surg, 4th edn → p328

High alcohol intake and other causes of chronic hepatocellular injury such as hepatitis B or C carriage are risk factors for the development of hepatocellular carcinoma. It is often multifocal and may arise on the background of pre-existing cirrhosis which can make the development of new signs more difficult to spot.

Chapter 8
Abdominal wall surgery

James Wood

It is all too easy to dismiss the abdominal wall when it comes to surgery and surgical diseases; it isn't a recognized organ or associated with any major speciality. It does, however, feature heavily in surgical examinations. The conditions of the abdominal wall are often chronic and commonplace and thus make an easy 'target' for clinical examinations. Understanding the principles of the diseases that afflict the abdominal wall and their assessment and treatment should mean that these sorts of clinical cases should be relatively 'easy money' when it comes to scoring marks in exams rather a trial.

The understanding of the principles of pathology and treatment rely heavily on the appreciation of the anatomy of the abdominal wall. Rather than 'run scared' because of this, some simple anatomy revision and practice questions should get all the key facts at your fingertips.

These questions will test both basic anatomy clinical features and principles of treatment and are typical of the way in which abdominal wall problems present and are tested in exams.

Neil Borley

QUESTIONS

Single Best Answers

1. Figure 8.1 shows several key landmarks in the right groin of a man. The bony prominences are labelled. The structure labelled A provides an important landmark in inguinal surgery.

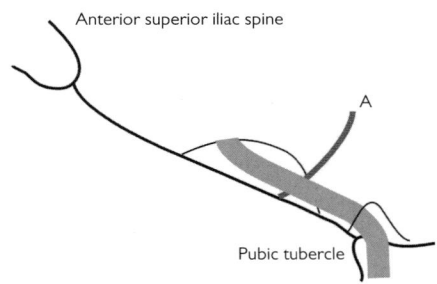

Anterior superior iliac spine

A

Pubic tubercle

Figure 8.1 Key landmarks in the right groin of a man

Which *single* term correctly describes structure A? ★

A Cremasteric artery

B External iliac artery

C Inferior epigastric artery

D Inferior pudendal artery

E Superficial circumflex artery

2. A 32-year-old man has a modest sized, freely reducible, indirect inguinal hernia. The hernia can be held in reduction by maintaining pressure over one particular location. Which *single* term most likely describes this location? ★

A Arcuate line

B Deep inguinal ring

C McBurney's point

D Mid-inguinal point

E Superficial inguinal ring

3. A 47-year-old woman has had a swelling in the right side of the abdomen for 2 months. A hernia is suspected and the lump's physical characteristics are being assessed. Which *single* clinical feature would confirm the clinical suspicion? ★

A Fluctuance

B Incompressibility

C Presence of fluid thrill

D Reduction on palpation

E Tenderness to palpation

4. An otherwise well 78-year-old woman has had a left groin lump for 2 months. A femoral hernia is suspected. There is a unilateral, reducible lump in the left femoral triangle with a cough impulse and thrill. Which is the *single* most appropriate piece of advice which should be given to the patient? ★★

A Discharge with advice to seek GP advice if symptoms occur

B Recommend an outpatient review in 3 months to assess hernia status

C Recommend investigation with groin ultrasound to confirm the diagnosis

D Recommend surgical exploration and repair within the next 6 weeks

E Recommend wearing a support truss

5. A 12-year-old boy has had a painful and swollen scrotum for 3h. There is no history of trauma, upper respiratory tract symptoms, or urinary symptoms. The testicle is very tender to palpation making clinical examination very difficult and unhelpful. Which is the *single* most appropriate next step? ★★★

A Arrange colour flow Doppler assessment

B Arrange for surgical exploration of the testicle

C Obtain a urine sample for urinalysis

D Prescribe IV analgesia and reassess

E Prescribe oral ciprofloxacin

Extended Matching Questions

Abdominal incisions

For each proposed operation choose the *single* most appropriate abdominal incision from the list of options. Each option may be used once, more than once, or not at all.

A Gridiron

B Groin

C Kocher right subcostal

D Lanz

E Lower midline

F Paramedian

G Pfannenstiel

H Rooftop

I Subumbilical

1. A 12-year-old boy undergoing an open excision of an appendix mass secondary to acute appendicitis. ★

2. A 28-year-old woman with acute lower abdominal pain suspected of a ruptured ovarian and undergoing a diagnostic procedure to confirm the diagnosis. ★★★

3. A 43-year-old woman undergoing hysterectomy for intermenstrual bleeding secondary to large uterine leiomyomas ('fibroids'). ★

4. A 55-year-old man with a past history of aortic aneurysm surgery undergoing elective open surgery for symptomatic gallstones. ★★★★

5. A 72-year-old man undergoing radical gastrectomy for gastric carcinoma. ★★★

Abdominal wall muscles

For each scenario choose the *single* most appropriate abdominal wall muscle from the list of options. Each option may be used once, more than once, or not at all.

A External oblique

B Iliacus

C Internal oblique

D Psoas major

E Pyramidalis

F Quadratus lumborum

G Rectus abdominis

H Transversus abdominis

I Serratus anterior

6. The muscle aponeurosis first encountered in the dissection during an open appendicectomy using a right iliac fossa incision. ★★★★

7. The muscle most likely to be involved with retroperitoneal abscess (e.g. retrocaecal abscess) formation. ★★

8. The muscle of the anterior abdominal wall which has muscle fibres running medially and superiorly. ★

9. The muscle with a thickened aponeurosis where it forms the inguinal ligament. ★★

10. The muscle that must be divided during surgical retroperitoneal approaches to the kidney. ★★★

ANSWERS

Single Best Answers

1. C ★　　　　OH Clin Surg, 4th edn → p338

This artery is the inferior epigastric artery. It originates from the external iliac artery (which passes laterally beneath the inguinal ligament to
become renamed as the common femoral artery). The inferior epigastric
artery marks the medial limit of those hernias appearing through the
deep ring which can be termed indirect. The cremasteric artery is one
of the three vessels present within the spermatic cord but is not visible
unless the cord is opened. The superficial circumflex artery is a branch
of the femoral artery running in the upper thigh. The inferior pudendal
artery is an artery of the perineum.

2. B ★　　　　OH Clin Surg, 4th edn → p338

Pressure at the deep inguinal ring will maintain reduction so long as the
defect is not very large. The deep ring is positioned at the mid-point of
the inguinal ligament. The femoral artery passes under the mid-inguinal
point which is mid-way between the pubis symphysis and the anterior
superior iliac spine and more medial than the deep ring; this also marks
the line of origin of the inferior epigastric artery. The superficial ring is
the exit of the inguinal canal just above and usually slightly medial to the
pubic tubercle.

McBurney's point is two-thirds along the line joining the umbilicus to the
anterior superior iliac spine and marks a common site for tenderness
in acute appendicitis. The arcuate line marks the lateral border of the
rectus sheath.

3. D ★　　　　OH Clin Surg, 4th edn → p346

There are numerous possibilities for an abdominal wall swelling.
Tenderness may indicate an acutely strangulated hernia but is also a
sign of an infected cyst or underlying infectious process appearing in the
abdominal wall. Fluctuance simply indicates a fluid filled structure and
is non-specific as is the presence of a fluid thrill which may occur with
bowel contents but also other fluid-filled structures such as a liquefied
haematoma or a seroma. Only a hernia will truly reduce on palpation
although intermuscular lipomas can become more difficult to locate on
palpation.

4. D ★★　　　　OH Clin Surg, 4th edn → p340

A femoral hernia is always a moderately high-risk hernia, especially so
in older females. Many present with acute symptoms or complications
and if the opportunity arises to deal with one when it is still asymptomatic it should be taken promptly. Investigation is only required if there

is considerable doubt over the diagnosis. Where this has been made clinically, there is no room for conservative management in patients otherwise fit for surgery as trusses are usually ineffective and review merely engenders the risk of acute complications.

5. B ★★★   OH Clin Surg, 4th edn → p350

This boy has torsion of the testis until proven otherwise. Although other less urgent diagnoses may be present (orchitis, acute hydrocoele, acutely symptomatic hernia), urgent surgical exploration is mandatory to reduce the risk of preventable infarction. Investigation such as Doppler assessment should not be used unless there has been a senior review since it risks delaying vital surgery. The seniors should be informed immediately even if that means interrupting them whilst they are operating.

Extended Matching Questions

1. A ★   OH Clin Surg, 4th edn → p82

The gridiron incision is the most appropriate incision for an open appendicectomy; it offers good exposure with a very low rate of complications such as hernia formation due to the approach via the muscle splitting. The Lanz incision is more generous and involves more muscle cutting. A midline incision is usually used only for complicated appendicitis or where the diagnosis is uncertain.

2. I ★★★   OH Clin Surg, 4th edn → p82

This woman is undergoing a diagnostic laparoscopy. Although several sites are commonly used for the establishment of a pneumoperitoneum and the first 10mm laparoscopic port, inferior to the umbilicus in the midline where the linea alba is relatively tethered and accessible is commonest and most useful here where a view of the pelvis is required. This is usually under direct vision or with the aid of a Veress needle.

3. G ★   OH Clin Surg, 4th edn → p82

This is a transverse incision and gives good access to the pelvis without needing to divide the lower abdominal muscles. It also offers the incision in one or two 'myotomes' which may make postoperative pain relief with locoregional anaesthesia more effective. Although a lower midline incision can be used it crosses more myotomes (thus is likely to be more painful) and is more prone to postoperative wound herniation.

4. C ★★★★   OH Clin Surg, 4th edn → p82

The Kocher incision is positioned in the right subcostal area. It provides good access for cholecystectomy or liver surgery and can be extended across the midline and laterally if major right upper quadrant access is required. The downside is that it involves substantial muscle division and is thus often painful.

5. H ★★★   OH Clin Surg, 4th edn → p82

At open surgery the rooftop incision provides good access for the abdominal dissection involved in any major open upper abdominal surgery including oesophageal, gastric, and liver surgery.

6. A ★★★★

The aponeurosis of external oblique is incised before encountering the internal oblique.

7. D ★★

Primary abscess formation can occur in the psoas muscles due to any retroperitoneal pathology (e.g. appendicitis, paraspinal abscess, perinephric abscess, retrosigmoid diverticular abscess).

8. C ★

Fibres of external oblique run medially and inferiorly (from chest wall to rectus sheath). Fibres of internal oblique run medially and superiorly (from iliac crest to rectus sheath).

9. A ★★

The external oblique at its inferior margin is thickened and in-rolled forming the inguinal ligament.

10. H ★★★

The retroperitoneal space is approached via the flank and thus the transversus abdominis muscle must be divided since it is the main muscle of the flank.

Chapter 9

Urological surgery

Simon Fisher

When the student contemplates potential causes of urinary tract obstruction, considering the anatomy of the drainage system from renal pelvis to urethral meatus and appreciation of potential causes of blockage will provide a useful diagnostic screen and will help one to review the breadth of conditions which may affect the renal tract. These include extrinsic compression, (for instance, due to retroperitoneal fibrosis or prostatic hypertrophy), mural involvement (infection, inflammation and transitional cell carcinoma), or luminal obstruction, (blood clot, stone, or valve). A firm grasp of appropriate investigations for urinary tract disease will aid diagnostic accuracy.

Urological surgery encompasses various aspects of neoplasia and developmental conditions. This chapter will test your knowledge of the presentation, diagnosis, management, and pathology of common urological malignancies including renal adenocarcinoma, transitional cell tumours, testicular tumours, and carcinoma of the prostate.

Urological conditions often occur in patients who may have other co-morbidities. Understanding the causes, investigation, and management of renal failure, appreciating the significance of haematuria, and knowing how to deal with an urological emergency of acute urinary obstruction will add to the medical student's or trainee surgeon's breadth of competence in general surgical practice.

Frank Smith

QUESTIONS

Single Best Answers

1. A 45-year-old man has severe colicky right-sided pain radiating from loin to groin, with nausea and vomiting. He is restless and tender in the right renal angle. Urinalysis shows blood +. Which is the *single* most appropriate investigation? ★★

A FBC, CRP, U&Es

B Intravenous urogram

C Plain abdominal X-ray (kidneys, ureter, bladder—KUB)

D Renal tract CT scan

E Renal ultrasound scan

2. A 60-year-old man is seen by the surgeon prior to discharge, following bilateral inguinal hernia repair earlier that day. He has worsening dull lower abdominal pain and distension. Prior to surgery he was fit and well. Which is the *single* most likely diagnosis? ★★

A Ilioinguinal nerve damage

B Scrotal haematoma

C Strangulated omental fat within repair

D Urinary retention

E Wound infection

3. A 58-year-old man has unremitting right-sided chest pain, worse on deep inspiration and coughing. He has urinary hesitancy, diminished stream, and post-micturition dribbling. He is tender in the right upper quadrant of the abdomen, and in the lower chest on palpation of the costal margin and lower ribs. His abdomen is soft. He has a hard enlarged prostate. His alkaline phosphatase is 260U/L. Which is the *single* most appropriate investigation? ★★

A Abdominal ultrasound

B Abdominal X-ray

C Chest X-ray

D Serum prostate-specific antigen

E Transrectal ultrasound scan

4. In clinic, the parents of a 5-year-old boy report that his foreskin often appears ballooned and appears to have a white tip. The boy's father had suffered from the same condition as a teenager. Which is the *single* most appropriate advice? ★★★★

A A course of antibiotics is required

B Foreskin biopsy should be undertaken

C The definitive treatment is circumcision

D The symptoms should settle without treatment

E Topical steroid ointment should be prescribed

5. A 66-year-old man has episodes of recurrent suprapubic pain, with haematuria and dysuria. He describes a poor urinary stream, difficulty in initiating micturition, and has to get up frequently during the night to void. Which is the *single* most likely diagnosis? ★

A Benign prostatic hyperplasia

B Bladder calculi

C Duplex system

D Neuropathic bladder

E Transitional cell carcinoma

6. A 51-year-old man has a painless persistent penile erection, unrelated to sexual stimulation, which has been present for some hours. Which *single* statement is most appropriate? ★★★★

A Aspiration of the corpora cavernosa is used to treat high-flow priapism

B High-flow priapism is commonly caused by blunt force trauma to the penis

C Low-flow priapism is characterized by involvement of the glans and corpus spongiosum

D Priapism involves damage to the tunica albuginea penis

E Serum electrophoresis to detect myeloma is diagnostic for high-flow priapism

7. A 30-year-old African-Caribbean man with sickle cell disease is seen in the emergency department with a persistent penile erection which has been present for 5h. His haemoglobin is 7.4g/dL. He has been started on IV fluids and supplementary oxygen. Which is the *single* next most appropriate management step? ★★★★

A Aspiration of the corpora cavernosa and manual pressure

B Blood transfusion

C Intracavernosal phenylephrine

D Oral beta-agonists

E Oral beta-antagonists

8. A 50-year-old stonemason develops erectile dysfunction. Which of the *single* points arising from his history is least likely to be related to his erectile problem? ★★★★

A He has a Dupuytren's contracture of his right palmar fascia

B He has become progressively deafer during the last 3 years

C He has had an inguinal hernia repair complicated by ilioinguinal nerve damage

D He reports that his GP is struggling to control his hypertension

E He suffered a slipped intervertebral disc at work last year

9. A 55-year-old man with type 2 diabetes has an inability to maintain an erection during intercourse. He reports morning erections. His only medication is for glycaemic control. He has a normal neurological examination. Which is the *single* most appropriate initial investigation? ★★★★

A Angiography

B Check blood HbA1c

C Check hormone profile (testosterone, FSH/luteinizing hormone, prolactin, thyroid function)

D Dynamic cavernosometry

E Psychological validated questionnaire

10. An ultrasound scan in a 50-year-old blind man with painless hae-maturia suggests the presence of adenocarcinoma of the kidney. A subsequent CT scan of his chest, abdomen, and pelvis confirms the diagnosis and shows renal vein invasion by the tumour (see Figure 9.1). The patient is anaemic but serum creatinine is 92μmol/L, potassium is 4.8mmol/L, calcium is 2.4mmol/L, and alkaline phosphatase is 33U/L.

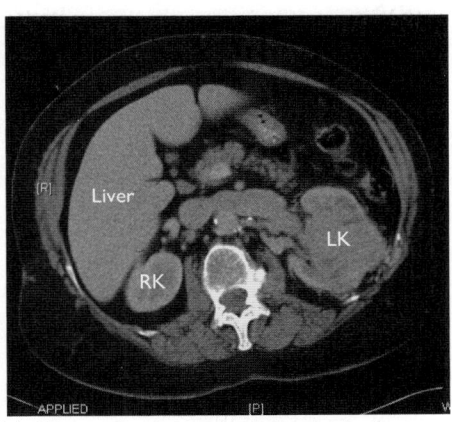

Figure 9.1 CT scan showing renal vein invasion by the tumour
Reproduced from Gardiner and Borley, *Oxford Specialty Training in Surgery*, 2009, with permission from Oxford University Press.

Which is the *single* most appropriate next step? ★★★★

A Biological (interferon/interleukin) therapy

B Genetic counselling

C Isotope bone scan

D Neoadjuvant chemotherapy

E Partial nephrectomy

11. A 45-year-old man develops a left scrotal mass with the appearance of distended tortuous veins. Scrotal and groin ultrasound confirms a varicocoele and a shrunken left testis (see Figure 9.2).

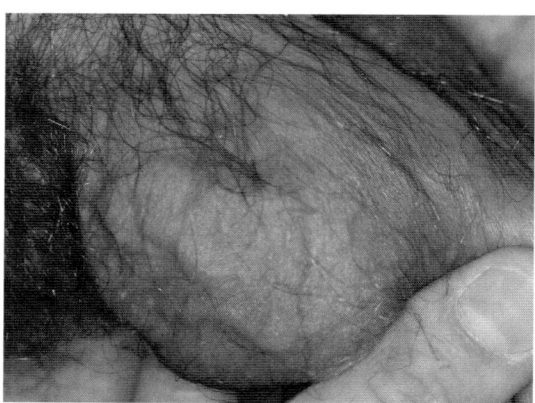

Figure 9.2 Ultrasound of the scrotum and groin confirming varicocoele and a shrunken left testis
Reproduced from Gardiner and Borley, *Oxford Specialty Training in Surgery*, 2009, with permission from Oxford University Press.

Which is the *single* most appropriate next step? ★★

A Interventional radiological embolization

B Intravenous urogram

C Renal ultrasound

D Sclerotherapy under local anaesthesia

E Surgical ligation

12. A 67-year-old man develops acute urinary retention after having painless haematuria for 3 months. Bladder irrigation has been established via a three-way catheter. Which is the *single* most appropriate next step in management? ★★★

A CT scan

B Flexible cystoscopy

C Rigid cystoscopy

D Ultrasound scan

E Urine cytology

13. A 70-year-old man, who worked in a petrochemical plant for many years, develops painless haematuria and undergoes transurethral endoscopic resection of an *in situ* transitional cell carcinoma of the bladder. Which is the *single* most appropriate next step in the patient's management? ★★★★

A Intravesical BCG

B Intravesical mitomycin C

C Partial cystectomy

D Radical cystectomy

E Regular check cystoscopy

14. A 93-year-old man has symptoms of prostatism, a craggy asymmetric prostate on rectal examination, and an elevated serum prostate-specific antigen. Transrectal ultrasound suggests the presence of a carcinoma localized to the prostate. Which is the *single* most appropriate next step in management? ★★★

A Active monitoring

B External beam radiotherapy

C Hormone therapy

D Radical prostatectomy

E Transurethral resection of prostate

15. A 13-year-old boy, who had mumps 4 months ago, develops sudden onset of pain in the right testicle, radiating to the right iliac fossa. He vomits twice. There is no tenderness or rebound on deep palpation of the abdomen. The right testicle is tender and high in the scrotum with a transverse lie. The patient is apyrexial, with white cell count 7×10^9/L. Which is the *single* most appropriate subsequent management? ★★

A Active observation

B Doppler assessment of testicular blood flow

C Measurement of viral titres

D Mid-stream urine and urethral swab

E Urgent surgical exploration of scrotum

16. A 25-year-old man notices a painless lump in his testicle on self-examination. An ultrasound scan confirms the presence of a testicular tumour. Tumour markers β-HCG and AFP are raised. A CT (see Figure 9.3) confirms the presence of lung metastases (stage 4 disease).

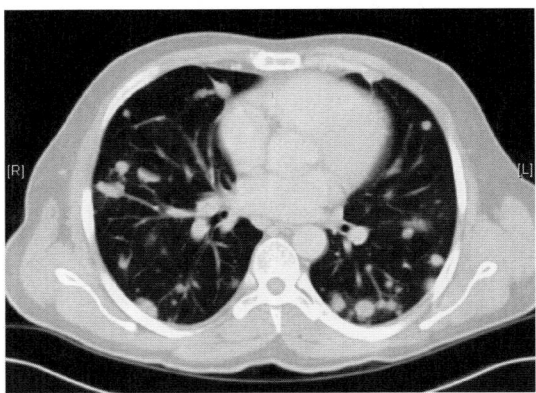

Figure 9.3 CT scan confirms the presence of lung metastases
Reproduced from Gardiner and Borley, *Oxford Specialty Training in Surgery*, 2009, with permission from Oxford University Press.

Which is the *single* most appropriate treatment for the likely tumour type? ★★★★

A Inguinal orchidectomy and chemotherapy

B Inguinal orchidectomy and radiotherapy

C Inguinal orchidectomy, retroperitoneal lymph node dissection and radiotherapy

D Transscrotal orchidectomy and chemotherapy

E Transscrotal orchidectomy and radiotherapy

17. A 38-year-old man is found to have an irregular, firm, non-transilluminating, painless testicular mass at an insurance medical examination. He has no other symptoms or signs. Which is the *single* most appropriate plan of investigation? ★★

A Testicular ultrasound scan; CT chest, abdomen

B Testicular ultrasound scan; CT chest, abdomen and brain

C Testicular ultrasound scan; CT chest, abdomen; and bone scan

D Testicular ultrasound scan; CT chest, abdomen, and brain; and bone scan

E Testicular ultrasound scan; serum β-HCG and AFP

18. During the night, a 69-year-old man with haematuria develops acute urinary retention and presents to the emergency department. He denies any trauma. Several attempts to pass a transurethral catheter have failed. Which is the *single* most appropriate initial management? ★★★

A Analgesia and check FBC, U&Es, creatinine

B Analgesia and fluid restriction

C Attempt to pass an irrigating three-way catheter

D Further attempt to pass single-lumen transurethral catheter

E Suprapubic catheterization

19. A 55-year-old woman develops constant right renal angle tenderness, worse on movement. Her temperature is 37.5°C; urine analysis demonstrates haematuria 1+ and white cells 1+, but no nitrites. Her white cell count is 12.3×10^9/L. Which is the *single* most appropriate initial investigation? ★★★

A Abdominal CT

B CT KUB

C Cystoscopy

D Intravenous urogram

E Renal ultrasound scan

20. A 42-year-old woman with type 1 diabetes develops groin and loin pain. Her temperature is 38.5°C. Examination reveals right renal angle and suprapubic tenderness. Her urine dip shows blood, nitrites, white cells, protein, and ketones. It has been sent for culture. Which is the *single* most appropriate next investigation? ★★★

A Arterial blood gases

B Blood cultures

C Blood glucose

D Renal tract ultrasound scan

E X-ray KUB

21. Nursing staff ask you to see a 65-year-old man, 6h following catheterization for retention, because he is producing 300mL of urine per hour. Which is the *single* most appropriate management? ★★★

A Check U&Es

B Check U&Es and clamp his catheter

C Check U&Es and consider IV fluids

D Check U&Es and restrict his oral fluids

E Check U&Es and stop bendroflumethiazide and angiotensin-converting enzyme inhibitor

22. A 47-year-old man develops sudden onset of colicky pain in his right loin, radiating into his testicle. The pain is severe and is associated with vomiting. A junior colleague asks for teaching about calculi. Which *single* statement with respect to urinary calculi is correct? ★★★

A Calcium phosphate stones are associated with renal tubular alkalosis

B Cystine stones are associated with urinary tract infection

C Staghorn calculi are associated with high urinary uric acid

D Struvite stones are the most common in UK patients

E There is seasonal variation in presentation of urinary tract lithiasis

Extended Matching Questions

Causes of scrotal swelling

For each scenario choose the *single* most likely cause from the list of options. Each option may be used once, more than once, or not at all.

A Epididymal cyst

B Epididymo-orchitis

C Hydrocoele

D Inguinal hernia

E Lipoma

F Non-seminomatous germ cell tumour

G Scrotal haematoma

H Seminoma

I Torsion of the hydatid of Morgagni

J Varicocoele

1. A 23-year-old man has a firm, painless irregular mass in his right testicle which has enlarged over 4 months. ★★

2. A 34-year-old man has a non-tender, fluctuant scrotal mass which causes discomfort when he wears tight pants. The scrotum transilluminates and the testis is not palpable. ★

3. A 45-year-old man has an intermittent lump in his left scrotum which is associated with groin discomfort. It is not possible to feel the upper limit of the mass within the scrotum. ★

4. A 37-year-old man notices a 1cm diameter lump in his scrotum which on examination is adjacent to, but feels separate from, the testicle. ★★★

5. A 62-year-old man has an acutely tender mass in the right side of his scrotum which has been associated with episodic dysuria during the previous 6 months. He is tender to testicular palpation and there is a mass adjacent to and apparently involving the testicle. ★★★

Causes of scrotal/testicular pain

For each scenario choose the *single* most likely cause from the list of options. Each option may be used once, more than once, or not at all.

A Epididymo-orchitis

B Glandular fever

C Mumps orchitis

D Ruptured testicle

E Scrotal haematoma

F Testicular torsion

G Testicular haematoma

H Thrombosed varicocoele

I Torsion of the hydatid of Morgagni

6. A 28-year-old man has scrotal pain in both testes, associated with a purulent urethral discharge. The pain is made marginally more comfortable by a scrotal support. ★★

7. A 16-year-old boy with maldescent of the testicle has sudden onset of right testicular pain. On palpation the testicle is in a high-lying position in the scrotum. ★

8. A 22-year-old man develops sudden onset of testicular pain. On transillumination of the scrotum there is the appearance of a localized dark region adjacent to the testicle. ★★

9. A 13-year-old boy has pain and swelling in his scrotum 24h after being hit by a cricket ball. ★★★

10. A 12-year-old boy with neck swelling develops a unilateral swollen tender testicle. ★★

Causes of haematuria/loin pain

For each scenario choose the *single* most likely cause from the list of options. Each option may be used once, more than once, or not at all.

A Bladder transitional cell carcinoma

B Glomerulonephritis

C Pelvic fracture

D Porphyria

E Prostate carcinoma

F Pyelonephritis

G Renal cell carcinoma

H Renal colic

I Schistosomiasis

11. A 35-year-old motorcyclist with bilateral fractured femurs has haematuria following a road traffic collision. There is blood at the penile meatus and a high-riding prostate on rectal examination. ★★

12. Painless haematuria, with frequency of micturition, in a 28-year-old man who spent 4 months trekking in Tanzania and Rwanda 1 year ago. FBC reveals an eosinophilia. ★★★★

13. Haematuria, weight loss, and mild renal angle tenderness in a 55-year-old woman with recent onset of back pain and white cell count of 5×10^9/L. ★★

14. A 45-year-old woman with type 1 diabetes and a history of recurrent urinary tract infections has microscopic haematuria, loin pain, and tenderness of the renal angle. Her temperature is 38.2°C and white cell count is 21×10^9/L. ★★

15. A 55-year-old man develops sudden onset of severe onset of colicky left loin pain radiating to the groin. Treatment with non-steroidal anti-inflammatory tablets and drinking several glasses of water appears to relieve the pain overnight. ★

ANSWERS

Single Best Answers

1. D ★★   OH Clin Surg, 4th edn → pp354, 358

Renal colic occurs in 3% of the population with a male predominance. The majority of stones are calcium (75%) or ammonium magnesium phosphate (15%) and are radio-opaque (90%). These may therefore be visible on KUB (C). However, CT is now the gold standard examination for imaging stones, replacing intravenous urogram which has the disadvantages of potentially causing contrast reactions and being unsuitable as a test in renal failure. Ultrasound may provide information about hydronephrosis but may miss small stones. A key management step is to identify those patients with infected, obstructed renal tracts by assessing for leucocytosis and high plasma creatinine. Common sites of renal stone impaction are shown in Figure 9.4. Occasionally ruptured abdominal aortic aneurysms, which occur most commonly in men aged over 65, may initially be confused with renal colic—beware the hypotensive patient with colic!

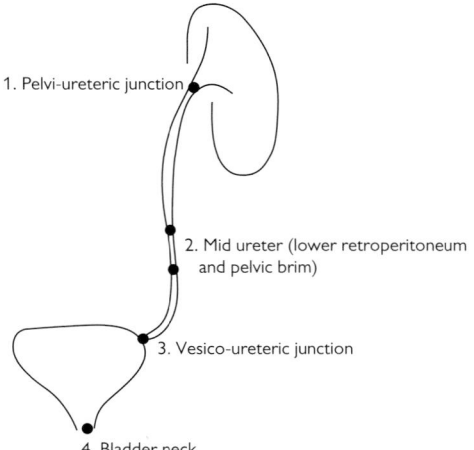

Figure 9.4 Common sites of renal stone impaction
Reproduced from McLatchie et al., *Oxford Handbook of Clinical Surgery*, 3rd edition, with permission from Oxford University Press.

2. D ★★   OH Clin Surg, 4th edn → p386

Acute urinary retention is a recognized complication of bilateral hernia repair and may be precipitated by pre-existing prostatic hypertrophy and anaesthetic drugs. If suspected, the diagnosis can be confirmed by examination in which there is a mass arising from the pelvis which one cannot get below on palpation and which is stony dull to percussion, and a bladder scan. Scrotal haematoma would be evident on examination. Wound infection would present later, ilioinguinal nerve damage presents as chronic pain, and omental fat strangulation within the repair is unlikely and would present as sharp pain.

3. C ★★   OH Clin Surg, 4th edn → p378

Chest X-ray is the most appropriate investigation in this case. This may help delineate any intrathoracic pathology and will demonstrate the skeletal prostatic carcinoma metastases in the ribs which are the source of this patient's pain. Abdominal ultrasound is not the appropriate investigation for bony pain. Prostate-specific antigen may be elevated following digital prostatic examination and is best employed as a screening test. Transrectal ultrasound will be valuable as a further investigation to image the prostate and facilitate biopsy. Pelvic MRI is employed to detect extracapsular spread and pelvic lymphadenopathy.

→ NICE guidelines on prostate cancer, 2008; http://guidance.nice.org.uk/CG58

4. C ★★★★   OH Clin Surg, 4th edn → p368

In childhood, physiological phimosis is identified by the lack of scarring at the preputial tip and by pouting of the inner layer of the foreskin upon attempted reduction. Lack of pouting and a white sclerotic tip characterize pathological phimosis, often secondary to balanitis xerotica obliterans. Physiological phimosis requires no treatment. Pathological phimosis may respond to steroid ointment but surgery, in the form of circumcision is the definitive treatment. Foreskin biopsy will be unhelpful and unnecessary in a 5-year-old. Antibiotics are not indicated unless there is an associated UTI.

5. A ★   OH Clin Surg, 4th edn → p362

Forty per cent of men over 60 years of age are affected by benign prostatic hyperplasia. It is the commonest cause of recurrent lower urinary tract infections, resulting in haematuria and dysuria. Haematuria associated with transitional cell carcinoma of the bladder, without secondary infection, is usually painless. B, C, and D do not present with the symptoms of bladder outflow obstruction described here. The International Prostate Symptom Score (IPSS) estimates the patient's perception of the severity of symptoms.

An online calculator is available at: → http://www.usrf.org/questionnaires/AUA_SymptomScore.html

→ Barry MJ, Fowler FJ Jr, O'Leary MP, et al. The American Urological Association symptom index for benign prostatic hyperplasia. The Measurement Committee of the American Urological Association. *J Urol* 1992; 148(5):1549–57.

6. B ★★★★   OH Clin Surg, 4th edn → p370

Priapism is painful persistent penile erection, unrelated to sexual stimulation. Low-flow priapism is caused by venous-occlusive congestion which results in secondarily reduced arterial inflow leading to hypoxia, acidosis, and hypercapnoea. It is characteristically painful and does not involve the glans and corpus spongiosum. Causes include drugs such as intracavernosal papaverine, prostacyclin, and psychotropics. Other causes include diseases such as myeloma and sickle cell, which result in abnormal blood viscosity, neurological and cerebrovascular disease, and local tumour infiltration. High-flow priapism is due to arteriocavernosal fistula, most commonly related to trauma and involves the glans and corpus spongiosum. It most commonly occurs due to blunt trauma to the penis or perineum. Peyronie's disease involves the tunica albuginea penis. Aspiration of the corpora cavernosa may be used to treat low-flow priapism.

7. B ★★★★   OH Clin Surg, 4th edn → p370

Sickle cell crisis is a systemic condition. Correcting any underlying anaemia improves global tissue oxygenation preventing hypoxic injury to other tissues and through this the priapism may also resolve. Subsequent measures include oral β-agonists, e.g. terbutaline, intracavernosal phenylephrine, and corpora cavernosa aspiration (up to 50mL) plus manual pressure.

8. C ★★★★   OH Clin Surg, 4th edn → p370

Dupuytren's contracture and tympanosclerosis are associated with Peyronie's disease, the formation of inelastic penile plaques resulting in damage to the tunica albuginea penis. This causes pain, deformity, and erectile dysfunction in one-third of sufferers. Neurological injury and anti-hypertensive drugs may also cause erectile dysfunction whereas damage to the ilioinguinal nerve is not implicated.

9. E ★★★★   OH Clin Surg, 4th edn → p372

The presence of morning erections is strongly indicative of a psychogenic cause. Specific validated questionnaires, e.g. The International Index of Erectile Function (IIEF-5) Questionnaire, have been developed for clinical practice. A check of hormone profile would then be appropriate if an organic cause was suspected. Dynamic cavernosometry would confirm a true vascular cause and only if revascularization was being considered would angiography be performed.

→ http://www.hiv.va.gov/provider/manual-primary-care/urology-tool2.asp

10. B ★★★★   OH Clin Surg, 4th edn → p374

Clinical evidence of neurological or ocular disease raises the possibility of von Hippel–Lindau disease, which is a dominantly inherited disease characterized by a defective gene on chromosome 3p25–26. Genetic counselling may facilitate screening of other family members. The only curative treatment for adenocarcinoma of the kidney is total nephrectomy; partial nephrectomy may be considered in small cancers (<4cm), located peripherally but would not be useful where there is renal vein invasion. These cancers are not chemosensitive. Radiotherapy is used to palliate bone metastases. Biological therapy may be used for metastatic disease but carries significant morbidity.

11. C ★★   OH Clin Surg, 4th edn → pp366, 374

It is important to exclude left renal adenocarcinoma with renal vein infiltration as a cause of obstructed drainage of the left testicular vein (one of its tributaries). Renal ultrasound should detect the tumour and is less invasive than an intravenous urogram. Sclerotherapy is not appropriate for varicocoeles. Symptomatic varicocoeles (causing pain, infertility or disrupted testicular growth) require treatment. Minimally invasive interventions are preferred, either embolization or surgical ligation which can be undertaken laparoscopically.

12. E ★★★   OH Clin Surg, 4th edn → p376

If malignancy is suspected urine cytology may show malignant cells and is non-invasive. Flexible cystoscopy with local anaesthetic gel will provide images of the bladder and urethra. Rigid cystoscopy (using an endoresectoscope) under general anaesthetic will allow lesion resection and histological diagnosis. Ultrasound allows assessment of pelvi-ureteric tumours. CT is required for local staging.

13. A ★★★★   OH Clin Surg, 4th edn → p376

Immunotherapy with intravesical BCG is effective in preventing progression to invasive transitional cell carcinoma in 60% of cases. Regular check cystoscopy is then required. Mitomycin C is used to treat superficial transitional cell tumours. Invasive transitional cell carcinoma, squamous cell carcinoma, and adenocarcinoma of the bladder are treated via radical cystectomy.

14. C ★★★   OH Clin Surg, 4th edn → p378

This man's life expectancy is less than 10 years, therefore management of his disease would be symptomatic control initially with hormonal (anti-androgen) therapy, possibly in combination with an alpha-blocker, and then if necessary via transurethral resection of prostate. Eighty per cent of prostatic carcinomas are androgen-dependent. In patients with a longer life expectancy, radical prostatectomy, external beam radiotherapy, or brachytherapy are treatment options. MRI is used to stage disease by assessing for extracapsular spread.

15. E ★★ OH Clin Surg, 4th edn → p366

The clinical findings suggest testicular torsion (see Figure 9.5). This is a surgical emergency and immediate surgical exploration is indicated. If the testis is viable then orchidopexy (fixing the testicle *in situ*) is undertaken. If the testicle is obviously not viable, orchidectomy is undertaken. The contralateral testicle should always undergo orchidopexy to prevent risk of future torsion. Duplex ultrasound may be useful in demonstrating blood flow, if immediately available, in equivocal cases, but surgery should not be postponed to wait for investigations. One-third of male adolescents with mumps develop acute epididymo-orchitis of which approximately 30% suffer testicular atrophy. Viral titres will not help diagnosis and the clinical findings are not suggestive of urinary tract infection.

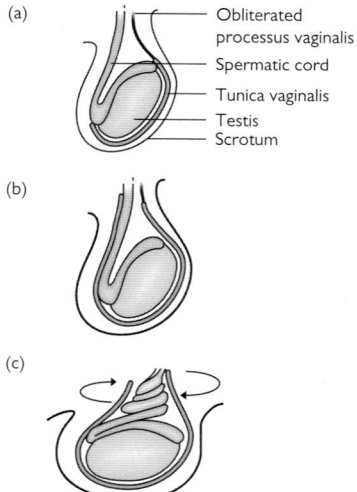

Figure 9.5 Testicular torsion
Reproduced from Gardiner and Borley, *Oxford Specialty Training in Surgery*, 2009, with permission from Oxford University Press.

16. A ★★★★ OH Clin Surg, 4th edn → p382

The tumour is likely to be a non-seminomatous germ cell tumour (NSGCT). These tumours, unlike seminomas, commonly undergo haematogenous spread and typically affect a younger age group of 20–30-year-old men. NSGCTs are chemosensitive and distant disease beyond the testis is treated by inguinal orchidectomy (with spermatic cord clamping to reduce the risk of tumour dissemination) and chemotherapy.

Retroperitoneal lymph node dissection is reserved for refractory nodal disease after this initial treatment. Transscrotal orchidectomy is inappropriate since resection of the spermatic cord and associated testicular lymphatic drainage is necessary at the deep inguinal ring.

17. A ★★   OH Clin Surg, 4th edn → p382

Testicular ultrasound will confirm the presence of the testicular tumour. Seminomas spread usually via the para-aortic lymph nodes to the chest. NSGCTs usually spread via the haematogenous route. NSGCT metastases are occasionally associated with a rise in serum β-HCG and AFP. CT chest, abdomen is required to stage disease. CT brain and bone scan are only performed if clinically indicated. Serum tumour markers may indicate metastatic disease and are helpful in determining response to treatment.

→ http://www.nice.org.uk/nicemedia/pdf/Urological_Manual.pdf

18. A ★★★   OH Clin Surg, 4th edn → p386

Whilst retention is painful, the significant potential complication is renal failure. Further attempts to pass a urethral catheter are unlikely to be successful and may result in a 'false passage'. Suprapubic catheterization is not advisable in the presence of haematuria in case the patient is bleeding from a bladder neoplasm, which may spread up the catheterization tract. Urological advice should be sought. In the presence of normal U&Es, an urologist would list the patient for 'next day' cystoscopy. Abnormal U&Es would prompt emergency cystoscopy.

19. E ★★★   OH Clin Surg, 4th edn → p374

This woman has pain which is not colicky in nature. It is disproportionate to her inflammatory response suggesting a non-infectious cause, which correlates with lack of nitrites in the urine. She is likely to have haemorrhaged into a cyst or tumour in the right kidney causing pain and mild inflammation. A suspicious ultrasound scan should be followed by CT.

20. C ★★★   OH Clin Surg, 4th edn → p356

This patient is septic from pyelonephritis and whilst she requires urgent antibiotics and blood cultures to exclude septicaemia, more significant is the ketonuria which may reflect a diabetic ketoacidosis. Renal tract ultrasound scan may be required later to investigate for renal abscess and abnormal anatomy underlying the pyelonephritis. Arterial blood gas would form part of her diabetic ketoacidosis work-up. KUB is not required.

21. C ★★★   OH Clin Surg, 4th edn → p386

This man probably has post-retention renal failure. It is important to ensure that his U&Es are normal to rule out a polyuric phase of renal failure. He may also need IV fluids to supplement oral intake and to ensure he remains euvolaemic. Stopping his diuretics may affect his cardiovascular co-morbidities. Clamping his catheter will result in retention. Oral fluid restriction may result in hypovolaemia.

22. E ★★★   OH Clin Surg, 4th edn → p358

Calcium phosphate stones are associated with renal tubular acidosis causing excessive calcium and phosphate secretion. Cystine stones (1–2%) are associated with cystinuria due to an autosomal recessive renal amino acid transport defect. Staghorn calculi have a high phosphate component and are associated with infection (see Figure 9.6). Struvite (triple phosphate—calcium, magnesium, ammonium) stones occur in approximately 10% of UK patients with renal tract lithiasis. Peak presentation of urinary stone disease occurs during the summer months, presumably due to increased levels of dehydration.

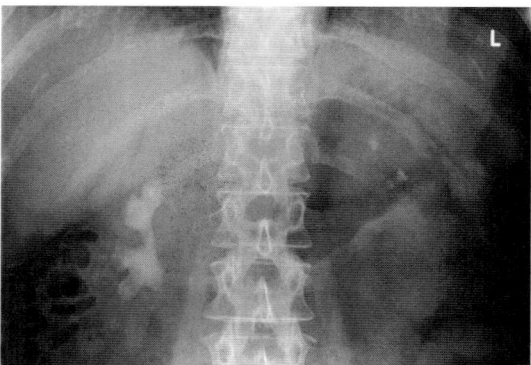

Figure 9.6 Staghorn calculi have a high phosphate component and are associated with infection
Reproduced from Gardiner and Borley, *Oxford Specialty Training in Surgery*, 2009, with permission from Oxford University Press.

Extended Matching Questions

1. F ★★

NSGCTs have a peak incidence in 20–30-year-olds whereas seminomas tend to occur in slightly older men in their 30s to 40s.

2. C ★

Transilluminable fluctuant scrotal mass. Hydrocoeles may be congenital (associated with a patent processus vaginalis; see Figure 9.7) or acquired. Hydrocoeles may occur acutely, secondary to intrascrotal pathology. Idiopathic hydrocoeles tend to be chronic.

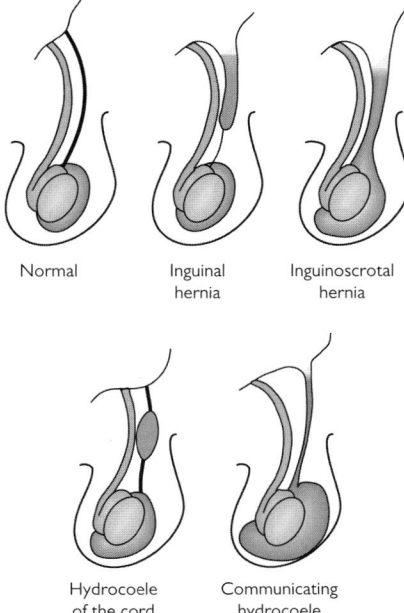

| Normal | Inguinal hernia | Inguinoscrotal hernia |

| Hydrocoele of the cord | Communicating hydrocoele |

Figure 9.7 Diagram showing different conditions arising from a patent processus vaginalis
Reproduced from Gardiner and Borley, *Oxford Specialty Training in Surgery*, 2009, with permission from Oxford University Press.

3. D ★

Classically, this mass is intermittent due to spontaneous reduction upon lying down due to the reduction in intra-abdominal pressure. The examiner cannot get above the mass as the hernia travels with the spermatic cord down through the superficial inguinal ring into the scrotum (see Figure 9.7).

4. A ★★★

This is a retention cyst in the epididymis which is separate to the testicle. The presence of an epididymal cyst can be confirmed by ultrasound. Cysts can be aspirated but may recur. Surgical excision risks loss of epididymal patency and recurrence and is best deferred until after childbearing age.

5. B ★★★

Epididymitis tends to occur by retrograde contamination by infected urethral contents via the vas deferens. This may spread to involve the testis. The inflammatory mass makes distinguishing testis and epididymis difficult. In men aged over 40, the commonest cause is bacterial infection which may be associated with urinary tract infections or prostatitis and is usually due to Gram-negative organisms. Sexually transmitted diseases may also be responsible but occur more frequently in men aged below 35.

6. A ★★

Epididymo-orchitis which may have occurred in association with a sexually transmitted infection or urinary tract infection. Relief of pain on scrotal elevation is Prehn's sign, distinguishing this condition from testicular torsion, although this is an inferior test compared to Doppler assessment of blood flow for the latter condition.

7. F ★

Testicular torsion which is associated with a high transverse ('bell-clapper') lie.

8. I ★★

Torted hydatid of Morgagni. The 'blue dot sign' is pathognomonic (when it occurs). The appendage is excised at scrotal exploration.

9. E ★★★

Scrotal haematoma. An ultrasound scan may be undertaken to determine the extent of any underlying testicular injury but this will be painful.

10. B ★★

Mumps orchitis. One-third of male adolescents with mumps develop orchitis, which is unilateral in 80%. In a third of these patients testes atrophy.

11. A ★★

This suggests pelvic fracture which may be associated with disruption of the urethra. Great care should be taken in catheterizing the patient so as not to risk further urethral damage.

12. I ★★★★

In this case the patient may have been infected by *Schistosoma haematobium*, which can be acquired even after short exposure such as swimming in freshwater lakes in Africa. Fork-tailed cercariae are liberated from the intermediate host, a species of freshwater snail. They penetrate the skin or mucus membranes of humans, the definitive host, forming schistosomulae which pass to lungs and liver and thence to the portal vein, before the mature worms migrate to the venules draining the pelvic viscera. Painless haematuria is the first and most common symptom. Frequency occurs due to later bladder neck obstruction.

13. G ★★

Haematogenous metastases to lungs and bone may cause respiratory symptoms, bone pain, or pathological fractures.

14. F ★★

The renal pelvis is inflamed and there may be small abscesses in the renal parenchyma. This is usually caused by organisms moving in a retrograde direction from the bladder. Differentiation from a perinephric abscess and to exclude obstruction should be made by early renal ultrasound as soon as possible. Adequate fluid administration and antibiotics are indicated.

15. G ★

This is probably an episode of renal colic which has resolved following passage of a small stone.

Chapter 10

Colorectal surgery

James Wood

Among the abdominal surgical specialities, colorectal surgery is, arguably, the most wide ranging. It spans a number of areas of practice each requiring many distinct knowledge bases. A large part of the speciality revolves around colorectal neoplasia which involves understanding of epidemiology, cell biology, and clinical genetics as well as appreciation of the major surgical presentations including some of the commoner abdominal emergencies, principles of surgical oncology, and pathology. Inflammatory bowel disease features a crossover area with medicine but all students of surgery need to understand the role of surgery in the context of advanced medical therapies including newer biological immunomodulatory treatments. On the other hand, functional pelvic floor disorders and diseases of the anal canal and rectum require understanding of anatomy and the wide range of local therapies available.

This chapter will test all these areas from pathology to anatomy, principles of major surgery, and outpatient treatments.

Neil Borley

QUESTIONS

Single Best Answers

1. A 23-year-old man presents with 6 weeks of increasingly frequent stools with blood-stained mucus mixed with diarrhoea. There is generalized mild abdominal tenderness but no guarding. Temperature is 37.6°C. Which is the *single* most likely diagnosis?★

A Crohn's disease

B Diverticular disease

C Haemorrhoids

D Rectal cancer

E Ulcerative colitis

2. A 24-year-old female undergoes a colonoscopy and is found to have multiple adenomatous polyps in the colon and rectum. Which is the *single* most likely genetic disorder to explain these findings? ★★★

A Gardner's syndrome

B Hereditary juvenile polyposis

C Lynch syndrome

D Peutz–Jeghers syndrome

E Sipple's syndrome

3. An isolated abnormality is seen in the descending colon during a colonoscopy to investigate 5 months of change in bowel habit and blood mixed with stools in a 72-year-old man. An image from the colonoscopy is shown in Figure 10.1. There is no family history of colorectal disease and he is otherwise fit and well. Biopsies are taken and the colonoscopy completed successfully.

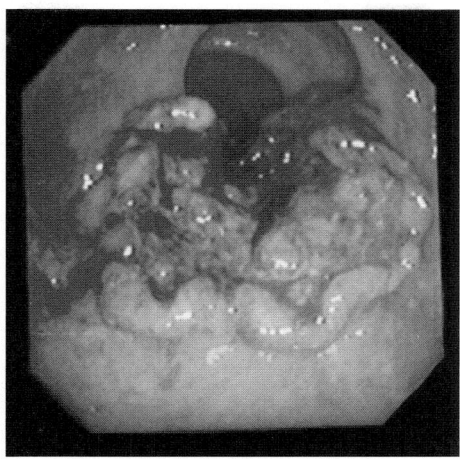

Figure 10.1 The colonoscopy shows an isolated abnormality

Which is the *single* most appropriate investigation that should be arranged next? ★★★★

A Chest X-ray

B CT scan of chest, abdomen, and pelvis

C Liver ultrasound scan

D MRI scan of the pelvis

E Whole body CT positron emission tomography scan

4. A 65-year-old man presents with rapid onset left iliac fossa pain and fever. He is tender in the left iliac fossa but there is no obvious palpable mass. Temperature is 37.7°C, pulse 84bpm, white cell count 14 × 10⁹/L, and CRP 54 mg/L. Which is the *single* most likely diagnosis? ★

A Acute appendicitis

B Sigmoid cancer

C Crohn's disease of the colon

D Acute sigmoid diverticulitis

E Ureteric colic

5. An 84-year-old woman has an 18-month history of intermittent swelling in the anus which appears when she strains to pass stools (see Figure 10.2).

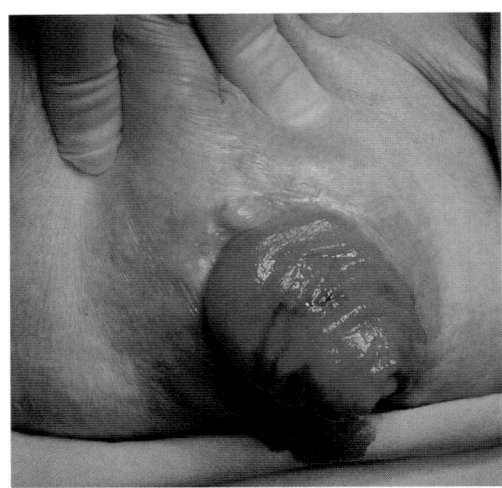

Figure 10.2 Swelling appears in the anus when she strains to pass stools

Which is the *single* most appropriate course of initial management? ★★★★

A Offer her a laparoscopic rectopexy

B Offer her banding of the excess mucosa

C Offer her Delorme's operation

D Recommend a course of injection sclerotherapy

E Recommend a course of stool softeners, and advice on bowel habit

6. A 34-year-old man has a red, tender, fluctuant swelling in his natal cleft with a swelling off to the left of the midline in the tissue of the left buttock. There are visible midline pits in the natal cleft. Which is the *single* most appropriate treatment? ★★★

A Fistulotomy under anaesthetic

B Incision and drainage under anaesthetic

C Oral antibiotics

D Wide excision and asymmetric natal cleft closure

E Wide excision and packing with daily dressings

7. A 28-year-old man has had a tender red swelling developing at his anal margin over 2 days. He has had recurrent episodes of similar symptoms with occasional discharge from the area. Examination reveals the external opening of a fistula in ano and an associated area of subcutaneous fluctuance. Which is the *single* most appropriate management plan? ★★

A Examination under general anaesthetic

B Immediate antibiotics and review in outpatients

C Incision and drainage on the ward

D MRI scan

E Needle aspiration on the ward

8. A 52-year-old man has several years' history of intermittent bright red blood on the toilet paper when defecation. There has been no mucus or change in bowel habit. Which is the *single* most appropriate first examination? ★★

A Colonoscopy

B CT colonography

C Endoanal ultrasound

D Flexible sigmoidoscopy

E Proctoscopy/rigid sigmoidoscopy

9. A 37-year-old woman has had sharp and persistent anal pain associated with defecation for 4 months. Occasionally, there are small amounts of blood on the toilet paper on wiping. There is a fissure present in the anal canal at the 6 o'clock position. Which is the *single* most appropriate treatment for her? ★★★

A Anal dilatation

B Botox injection

C Diltiazem cream

D Lateral internal sphincterotomy

E Prednisolone suppositories

10. A 73-year-old woman has had sudden onset of acute profuse rectal bleeding 4h ago. She has had no abdominal pain. The pulse rate is 105bpm, blood pressure of 95/50mmHg, capillary refill time is 5sec and oxygen saturations are 96% on supplemental oxygen via a non-re-breathing reservoir. Which is the *single* most appropriate first step in her management? ★

A Catheterize the patient

B Insert two large bore cannulae

C Organize flexible sigmoidoscopy

D Organize rigid sigmoidoscopy

E Organize mesenteric angiogram

11. A 78-year-old man who is known to have sigmoid diverticular disease has developed left lower quadrant pain over the last 8 days with 48h of constant severe pain, feeling febrile with sweating episodes and shakes. His temperature is fluctuating up to 39.2°C, the pulse is 84bpm, blood pressure 125/74mmHg, and there is localized tenderness in the left lower quadrant but no generalized guarding or tenderness. Intravenous fluids and antibiotics are started. An urgent CT scan of the pelvis is shown in Figure 10.3.

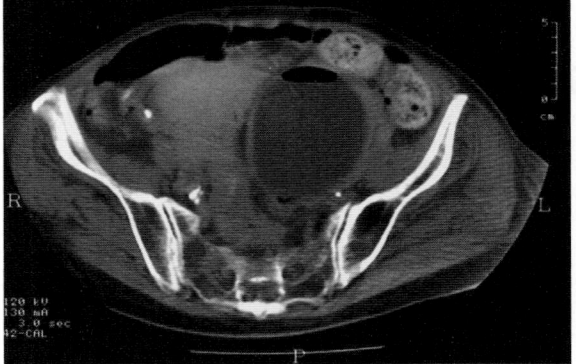

Figure 10.3 An urgent CT scan shows this appearance in the pelvis

Which is the *single* most appropriate treatment he should be offered? ★★★

A Formation of a defunctioning loop colostomy

B Colonoscopy and colonic stent insertion

C Continued IV antibiotics and close monitoring

D CT guided drainage

E Sigmoid colectomy and end colostomy (Hartmann's procedure)

12. A 74-year-old man who had a right hemicolectomy 5 days ago is now unwell with shortness of breath, generalized abdominal pain and mild distension. Temperature is 37.8°C, pulse 102bpm and blood pressure 127/67mmHg. There is generalized abdominal tenderness with involuntary guarding on the left side. He is being given supplemental oxygen and has intravenous 0.9% saline running. Which is the *single* most appropriate first step you should take? ★★★

A Administer IV antibiotics

B Arrange an abdominopelvic CT scan

C Arrange an emergency laparotomy

D Request an erect chest X-ray

E Request an ultrasound scan and radiological drain

Extended Matching Questions

Abdominal masses

For each scenario choose the *single* most likely abdominal mass from the list of options. Each option may be used once, more than once, or not at all.

A Appendix mass
B Colonic carcinoma
C Diverticular abscess
D Femoral hernia
E Inguinal hernia
F Lymphoma
G Palpable bladder
H Pelvic abscess
I Renal transplant

1. A 65-year-old diabetic man has a painless, smooth, firm mass in the right iliac fossa. He also has a radiocephalic fistula. ★★

2. A 75-year-old woman has a haemoglobin of 9.8g/dL, mean corpuscular volume of 72fL, and ferritin of 6mcg/L. There is a palpable mass in the right iliac fossa. ★★★

3. A 10-year-old boy with 1 week of vague abdominal pains, 24h of a swinging pyrexia, and a tender, firm mass in the right iliac fossa. ★★★

4. A 75-year-old woman with 48h of vomiting, abdominal distension, and a new swelling in the left groin which appears to arise below the inguinal ligament. ★

5. A 70-year-old man with 5 weeks of intermittent left iliac fossa pain, anorexia, and anergia. He has lost 2kg of weight. He has had low-grade fevers for the last 3 nights. There is a tender mass in the left lower quadrant. ★★★★

Investigation of colorectal complaints

For each scenario choose the *single* most appropriate first investigation from the list of options. Each option may be used once, more than once, or not at all.

A Barium enema (double contrast)

B Colonoscopy

C CT scan of the abdomen and pelvis

D Endoanal ultrasound scan

E Flexible sigmoidoscopy

F Plain abdominal X-ray

G MRI scan of the abdomen

H Transabdominal pelvic ultrasound scan

I CT colonography

6. A 76-year-old man with a haemoglobin of 7.9g/dL, mean corpuscular volume of 72fL, and mean corpuscular haemoglobin of 32pg found on routine bloods tests during a GP medical check. ★★★★

7. A 72-year-old woman with 3 months of change in bowel habit including frequent diarrhoea and urgency but no blood in the stool. Her weight is stable and there are no masses palpable. ★★★

8. A 68-year-old man with 10 days of progressive abdominal distension, colicky pains, reduced bowel frequency, and 24h of vomiting. ★

9. A 48-year-old woman with 8 months of intermittent, bright red rectal bleeding seen on the toilet paper associated with defecation. The anus and rectum are normal to examination. ★★

10. A 32-year-old woman with a 6-month history of pelvic discomfort and pressure in the rectum. Bowel habit has been unchanged. There is no abdominal mass and no rectal abnormalities palpable. ★★★★

Colorectal anatomy

For each scenario choose the *single* most likely anatomical location for the site of the pathology from the list of options given in Figure 10.4. Each option may be used once, more than once, or not at all.

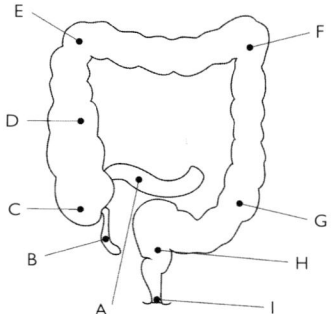

Figure 10.4 Colorectal anatomy

11. A 57-year-old man smokes 20 cigarettes per day and suffers from hypertension and ischaemic heart disease. He has had 2 days of left-sided abdominal pain and distension with 12 hours of passing dark, bloody loose stools. There is left-sided abdominal tenderness, his temperature is 37.7°C. ★★★

12. A 42-year-old man with bright red rectal bleeding on the toilet paper during and after defecation for 3 years who has noticed mucus discharge per rectum on his underwear. His bowel habit is unchanged and there has been no abdominal pain. ★★

13. A 24-year-old woman with lower abdominal pains and loose stools increasing in frequency over 18 months with 4kg weight loss. Stools are poorly formed with no blood or mucus. There is the presence of a fullness in the lower abdomen. ★★

14. A 66-year-old man with 3 months of worsening frequency of bowel action, lower abdominal pain, and bloating. He has had 3 days of abdominal distension and colicky pain. Temperature is 38.1°C, white blood cell count is 13.4 × 10⁹/L, and CRP is 48mg/L. ★

15. An 82-year-old woman underwent external beam radiotherapy for the treatment of carcinoma of the cervix 5 years ago. For 3 years she has had the passage of mucus and blood with some clots per rectum which occurs mostly during defecation. She has developed the passage of flatus and faecal matter per vagina over the last 2 months. ★★★★

ANSWERS

Single Best Answers

1. E ★   OH Clin Surg, 4th edn → p392

This is a classic presentation for ulcerative colitis: the key features are frequency (due to colonic involvement), bloody mucus, urgency (due to rectal hypersensitivity), and diarrhoea. Rectal cancer and diverticular disease typically present in the ageing population although both can be seen as young as patients in their 20s. The bleeding associated with rectal cancer is often smaller volume and mixed with normal looking stools whilst that of diverticular disease (as distinct from acute diverticulitis) is commonly episodic frank blood per rectum. Crohn's disease can cause diarrhoea but is less commonly associated with blood in stools. Haemorrhoids can cause bright red rectal bleeding but not typically diarrhoea or mucus.

2. A ★★★   OH Clin Surg, 4th edn → p399

This lady most likely has a multiple adenomatous polyp syndrome. Juvenile polyps are mucinous and not adenomatous although may be diagnosed in young adults. Similarly the polyps of Peutz–Jeghers syndrome are hamartomatous with a characteristic proliferation of smooth muscle in their core. Both these syndromes can increase the risk of colorectal carcinoma. Lynch syndrome is the name for hereditary non-polyposis colon carcinoma and Sipple's syndrome is one form of inherited multiple endocrine neoplasia. Gardner's syndrome is a variant of familial adenomatous polyposis with the additional presence of osteomata and fibrous bone cysts.

3. B ★★★★   OH Clin Surg, 4th edn → p400

This is a colonic carcinoma; the centre is ulcerated and bleeding freely. The biopsies should confirm the diagnosis. The main issues are (1) to assess for the presence of distant disease and (2) to assess if the primary could be surgically removed. The most likely organs for colorectal cancer to metastasize to are the liver and lungs. Liver ultrasound may be used to evaluate abnormalities seen on CT scanning but is limited only to the liver in extent. A CT positron emission tomography scan is a useful examination to assess for occult metastatic disease or where contrast-enhanced CT scanning is equivocal but is not routinely used as first-line investigation. Chest X-ray is very insensitive for small pulmonary abnormalities and has been completely replaced by thoracic CT scanning. Thus CT scanning of the chest, abdomen, and pelvis is the ideal first and often only staging investigation. A pelvic MRI scan is concerned with assessing local spread of rectal cancers.

4. D ★ OH Clin Surg, 4th edn → p404

This is a common presenting complaint to the acute surgical take team. Diverticula commonly occur in the sigmoid colon and when they become inflamed (diverticulitis) they cause left iliac fossa pain, tenderness, and fever.

A perforated cancer may simulate diverticulitis but it is less common and a palpable mass is usual. An acute presentation of colonic Crohn's disease would be very rare at this age and ureteric colic would not be associated with fever unless complicated by ascending infection.

5. E ★★★★ OH Clin Surg, 4th edn → p407

The appearance is typical of a full thickness rectal prolapse. It is too large and cylindrical to be simple mucosal prolapse. Thus injection sclerotherapy and banding are both inappropriate. Although a rectopexy (fixation of the rectum) or a Delorme's procedure (mucosal excision and plication) are treatments for prolapse, and can be very effective, the mainstay of initial treatment is proper assessment and dealing with the underlying cause of the prolapse, which is inappropriate straining especially if the stools are hard.

6. B ★★★ OH Clin Surg, 4th edn → p408

This is a pilonidal abscess. It may be mistaken for a perianal abscess or a fistula in ano but the presence of the midline pits and the disease process located in the natal cleft are almost diagnostic. Pilonidal abscesses occur superior to the perianal area in the natal cleft between the buttocks. Early infection where there is no suppuration may be treated by oral antibiotics but here there is a fluctuant swelling indicating an underlying abscess so incision and drainage is required although that is usually followed up with antibiotics. Wide excision either with or without primary closure is a definitive treatment for pilonidal sinus disease but is best not undertaken where there is active sepsis which should be dealt with first.

7. A ★★ OH Clin Surg, 4th edn → p410

This man most likely has a perianal abscess. This will require examination under general anaesthetic with incision and drainage although he should ideally be consented for appropriate management of a fistula if it is found. It is usually too painful to do this properly on the ward and the underlying fistula will be missed if you do. Simple aspiration is inadequate. MRI scanning may be helpful for complex perianal fistulae or recurrent abscesses where surgery has failed to find the infection or fistula.

8. E ★★   OH Clin Surg, 4th edn → p412

This man most likely has haemorrhoids causing his bleeding. In the clinic proctoscopy and rigid sigmoidoscopy can be performed to make the diagnosis. Although a flexible sigmoidoscopy may be used to exclude any other diagnoses the simple clinic tests should be done to try to confirm the clinical suspicion. Colonoscopy or CT colonography would only be indicated if another pathology was found at rigid sigmoidoscopy or if there was an extensive family history of colorectal neoplasia.

9. C ★★★   OH Clin Surg, 4th edn → p414

This is a simple fissure in ano. There is no reason to suspect an alternative or underlying diagnosis. Unless it fails to respond to first-line treatment further investigation under anaesthetic is not necessary and treatment should be started first. It is thought that the pathogenesis of anal fissures involve spasm of the internal anal sphincter with associated changes in anal blood flow and poor healing. Most cases of anal fissure will heal provided the pressure within the anal canal can be reduced, likely through improving anocutaneous blood flow. Any of the first four treatments will achieve that reduction but the one with the lowest risk of side effects is diltiazem ointment. Diltiazem causes smooth muscle relaxation and helps to decrease the spasm. Anal dilatation is an outdated treatment which can cause faecal incontinence due to uncontrolled stretching of the anal sphincter. Botox injection and lateral sphincterotomy are usually reserved for cases which do not respond to topical treatment. Predsol will do little to improve the fissure and may delay healing.

10. B ★   OH Clin Surg, 4th edn → p416

This patient requires resuscitation in the first instance. Depending on the quantity of blood loss the patient may require significant fluid replacement and transfusion. Catheterization may be useful to monitor the urine output in an unstable patient but the first step is to establish access and give IV fluids. Investigations can take place after resuscitation has been fully initiated.

11. D ★★★   OH Clin Surg, 4th edn → p404

There is an obvious well-formed abscess to the left side of the image with fluid and gas in it. This is typical for a diverticular abscess and fits with the clinical picture. There is no clinical evidence for the presence of widespread intra-abdominal infection so emergency operation and resection is not mandatory and ideally should be avoided in an elderly patient. A diverting loop stoma of any kind will not deal with the established abscess and neither will simple continued antibiotic therapy although the antibiotics must be continued with drainage. Drainage of the abscess is required and if this can be achieved by radiological guided methods this is ideal. Surgery, either drainage or resection should be reserved for failure of radiological drainage.

A colonic stent would only be applicable if there was obstruction without any evidence of infection since there is a risk of damage to the wall of the colon during insertion.

12. A ★★★   OH Clin Surg, 4th edn → p420

In this clinical setting it must be assumed that the patient has an anastomotic leak. Five days is a typical length of time after surgery for this to happen. The vague abdominal signs and left-sided tenderness should not dissuade you from this diagnosis. A CT scan is the best investigation to confirm the diagnosis if the patient is stable enough and for those who are acutely unwell a prompt return to theatre for surgery is often appropriate. A minor leak with a contained collection might be identified by scan and a radiological drain placed but for all these courses of action infection is the predominant issue. The first step should always be resuscitation and IV antibiotics whilst the other plans are being made according to the status of the patient.

Extended Matching Questions

1. I ★★

The radiocephalic fistula indicates that this patient has had haemodialysis. The fact that the mass is painless and non-tender effectively excludes inflammatory or septic causes. A chronically distended bladder may be asymptomatic but would be more likely palpable in the midline. A mass in the iliac fossae is likely to be a transplanted kidney.

2. B ★★★

Colonic carcinoma, especially right-sided lesions such as in the caecum, is a common cause of iron deficiency anaemia (confirmed by the low ferritin level). Lymphoma may cause anaemia but not usually of an iron deficient pattern.

3. A ★★★

At his age, this boy has most likely had appendicitis which has now developed into an abscess. Appendicitis does not always present with classic symptoms and signs. Diverticulitis may present with a right-sided mass of symptoms but it is rare and exceptionally so at this age. A pelvic abscess may result from appendicitis, especially after surgical treatment but it is usually impalpable and diagnosed on CT or ultrasound imaging.

4. D ★

The clinical features are of intestinal obstruction. The location of the mass below the inguinal ligament makes an intra-abdominal cause such as diverticular disease very unlikely. It is difficult to be certain whether an apparent hernial mass is truly arising below the inguinal ligament, the age and sex of the patient make a femoral hernia more likely as does the presentation (50% of femoral hernias present for the first time urgently with obstructive symptoms).

5. C ★★★★

The clinical features are of a septic process. Lymphoma may be suggested by the apparent night sweats but these may also be due to a collection within the abdomen or pelvis and the short history of night sweats is against a diagnosis of lymphoma. A locally perforated colonic carcinoma might give symptoms such as these but at his age an abscess related to diverticular disease is more likely.

6. B ★★★★

This man is most likely to have an iron deficiency anaemia although ideally a serum ferritin should be performed to check that there is proven iron deficiency. The most likely causes in the lower GI tract are a proximal colonic carcinoma or large adenoma, colitis, or recurrent anorectal bleeding causes such as haemorrhoids. Although barium enema and CT colonoscopy would both be likely to locate the pathology, neither would be able to confirm the diagnosis by biopsy so the best test is a colonoscopy. The other two would be more likely used in patients unfit for colonoscopy.

7. B ★★★

A change in bowel habit requires investigation of the whole large bowel. Although most patients are concerned that the diagnosis may be related to a tumour, colorectal inflammation such as colitis of one form or another may be the cause. Colonoscopy is the only examination which allows both inspection of the colon and biopsies to be taken if no focal lesions are found.

8. C ★

The symptoms here suggest intestinal obstruction. Although a plain abdominal X-ray may well suggest obstruction, an abdominal CT scan is more likely to confirm the diagnosis and may well suggest the underlying pathology which may help decisions on how to manage the patient. Any investigations which require the administration of bowel preparation, including colonoscopy, CT colonography, and barium enema are contraindicated until the presence of obstruction has been assessed by CT scan and a flexible sigmoidoscopy may not reach the level of any pathology causing the symptoms.

9. E ★★

Bright red rectal bleeding usually arises from the rectum or sigmoid colon. A flexible sigmoidoscopy examines the rectum, sigmoid, and usually the descending colon to the splenic flexure. A colonoscopy would assess the same area as well as the rest of the colon but is associated with an increased risk of complications compared to flexible sigmoidoscopy.

10. H ★★★★

The symptoms suggest a pelvic mass. Investigations to assess the rectum or large bowel such as flexible sigmoidoscopy, colonoscopy, and barium enema may assess the large bowel but would not diagnose a pelvic mass. CT scanning would make the diagnosis but in a young woman would best be avoided and a non-ionizing investigation used as first line. MRI of the abdomen is not ideal for assessment of the pelvis. Ultrasound scanning is not associated with any risk and is non-invasive with high sensitivity for detecting a pelvic mass.

11. F ★★★   OH Clin Surg, 4th edn → p396

The history is suggestive of ischaemic colitis. The background risk factors and the development of bloody stools with pain and abdominal tenderness are typical. Acute diverticulitis is possible but the dark bloody stools are more suggestive of ischaemia. The commonest site for ischaemia is where the colonic blood supply is poorest and this is where the marginal artery from the middle colic artery and the upper branches of the left colic artery link up which is around the splenic flexure.

12. I ★★   OH Clin Surg, 4th edn → p416

These symptoms point to an anorectal cause for the bleeding. Although bright red rectal bleeding can originate from the rectum and left colon, it is more likely that it would be mixed in with the stools rather than on the surface of the stools. The mucus could arise from a rectal cause but as it is soiling the underwear it is most likely from the anus. The pathology cannot be confidently predicted from the clinical features but haemorrhoids remain the single most likely diagnosis.

13. F ★★   OH Clin Surg, 4th edn → p394

The features of loose stools and frequency suggest a form of inflammatory bowel disease. Colitis of one form or another or Crohn's disease are both possible but the absence of blood in the stools makes colitis less likely. The associated weight loss is typical for Crohn's disease. Crohn's may affect any part of the colon or small bowel but the terminal ileum is most likely and the presence of lower abdominal fullness supports this.

14. G ★   OH Clin Surg, 4th edn → p402

The history of change in bowel habit and lower abdominal pain suggests lower colonic pathology. Change in bowel habit is much less common with right-sided pathology. The presence of new features of colonic obstruction (distension and colicky pain) coupled with the features of inflammation are most typical for diverticulitis which most commonly affects the sigmoid colon although it can affect anywhere in the colon. It is impossible to exclude a carcinoma as the cause but the clinical pattern strongly suggests pathology in the sigmoid colon.

15. H ★★★★   OH Clin Surg, 4th edn → p396

The symptoms of faeces and wind per vagina indicate the presence of an enterovaginal fistula which could originate from anywhere in the bowel. However, the terminal ileum, sigmoid, and rectum are the most likely originating sites, given their position in the pelvis. The fact that she did not undergo hysterectomy means that the upper sigmoid and other loop of bowel are less likely to be present next to the vaginal wall tissue. Diverticular disease, Crohn's disease, and colorectal cancer could all be a cause but the passage of blood and mucus per rectum for 3 years is typical of radiation-induced damage to the rectum ('radiation proctitis'). One complication of this is the development of a spontaneous rectovaginal fistula.

Chapter 11

Paediatric surgery

Simon Fisher

Understanding that children are not small adults, and that they come in different sizes and stages of development, is fundamental to paediatric surgery. Knowledge of a child's weight is crucial when considering fluid and medication administration.

Moreover, babies have immature physiology and less functional reserve compared to older children. Understanding basic embryology will unravel some of the mysteries of developmental pathology encountered by the paediatric surgeon, such as oesophageal atresia, malrotation of the gut, annular pancreas, and maldescent of the testis.

The paediatric surgeon deals with some of the same surgical conditions that affect adults, but even management of a common condition such as inguinal hernia, has different therapeutic implications in children and adults. Paediatric surgery demands gentle tissue handling and delicate technique. Good communication skills are a prerequisite for dealing with the distraught or ill child and anxious parents, and the surgeon often retains a clinical interest in his or her patient, well into young adulthood.

This chapter will test your knowledge of principles of surgical management of sick children and your understanding of presentations of some of the more commonplace conditions encountered by surgeons in this demanding, yet rewarding, discipline.

Frank Smith

QUESTIONS

Single Best Answers

1. A 3-day-old baby whose mother had polyhydramnios during pregnancy is noted to have feeding problems. Nursing staff report that the baby becomes distressed during feeding, starts choking, turns blue, and then regurgitates the feed. You notice the baby drooling. Which is the *single* most likely diagnosis? ★★

A Annular pancreas

B Duodenal atresia

C Oesophageal atresia

D Pharyngeal pouch

E Pyloric stenosis

2. A 2-day-old baby appears distressed and has bile-stained vomiting with passage of a small amount of blood per rectum. A plain abdominal X-ray shows abnormal gas patterns with dilated small bowel and duplex ultrasound scan of the abdomen demonstrates a reversed relationship between superior mesenteric vein and artery. Which is the next *single* most appropriate step? ★★★

A Barium meal

B Barium enema

C Exploratory laparotomy

D Insert nasogastric tube and reassess at 24h

E Laparotomy and small bowel resection

3. A neonate weighing 3.5kg, with vomiting and dehydration, needs fluid replacement. A junior medical student asks about the rationale for planning the fluid resuscitation. Which *single* statement is correct? ★★★

A He requires approximately 1mmol/kg of potassium per day in solution

B He should be given IV maintenance fluid at a rate of approximately 4mL/kg/h

C His blood volume is approximately 40mL/kg

D His normal oral fluid intake should be approximately 50mL/kg/day

E His normal systolic blood pressure is approximately 80mmHg

4. A 5-week-old boy is brought to clinic by his mother who has noticed that he has developed forceful vomiting after every feed. He appears dehydrated. Which is the *single* most likely collection of electrolyte disturbances that this condition is likely to be associated with? ★★

A Hyperkalaemic hypochloraemic alkalosis

B Hypokalaemic hyperchloraemic acidosis

C Hypokalaemic hyperchloraemic alkalosis

D Hypokalaemic hypochloraemic acidosis

E Hypokalaemic hypochloraemic alkalosis

5. A 3-day-old boy on the neonatal ward has had bilious vomiting from birth and has epigastric fullness on examination. A supine plain abdominal X-ray reveals gas in the stomach and first part of the duodenum (see Figure 11.1).

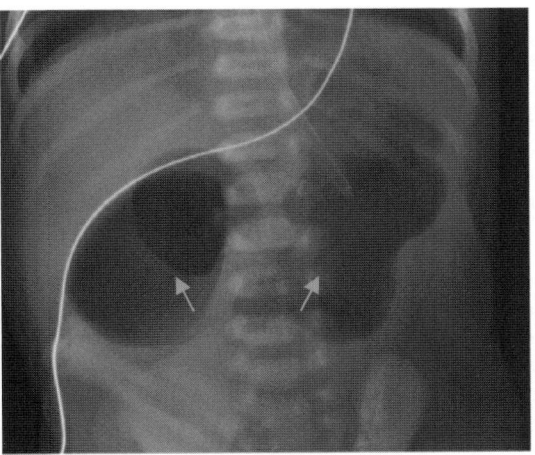

Figure 11.1 The X-ray reveals gas in the stomach and the first part of the duodenum
Reproduced from Gardiner and Borley, *Oxford Specialty Training in Surgery*, 2009, with permission from Oxford University Press.

Which is the *single* most likely diagnosis? ★★

A Biliary atresia

B Duodenal atresia

C Jejuno-ileal atresia

D Pancreas divisum

E Pyloric stenosis

6. A 6-month-old boy is brought to the GP by his parents, who have noticed when bathing him that he does not appear to have a palpable testis in the left side of his scrotum. A medical student asks about the condition and its management. Which *single* statement is correct? ★★

A A retractile testis should be fixed in the scrotum at 1–2 years

B Absence of a scrotal testis is more commonly due to agenesis than arrested descent

C An intra-abdominal testis is associated with a fourfold increased risk of testicular cancer

D An undescended testis occurs in approximately 10% of newborn boys

E Torsion is a common presentation of incomplete testicular descent

7. A 7-month-old boy is brought to the paediatric emergency department by his mother, with intermittent abdominal pain, abdominal distension, and vomiting. His mother reports that he is passing bright red jelly-like stools. There is no evidence of shock or peritonism but he has a sausage-shaped mass in the right upper quadrant. Which is the *single* most appropriate diagnostic test? ★★

A Air contrast enema

B Barium contrast enema

C CT abdomen and pelvis

D Diatrizoic acid contrast enema

E Ultrasound scan of the abdomen

8. A 3-day-old baby is vomiting and has a right iliac fossa mass. The ward nurses report that the baby has yet to pass meconium. 'Bright spots' were seen in the child's bowel at antenatal ultrasound scan. Which is the *single* most likely diagnosis? ★

A Anorectal malformation

B Cystic fibrosis

C Hirschsprung's disease

D Intussusception

E Jejuno-ileal atresia

9. The parents of a 1-year-old boy are anxious that they cannot retract his foreskin when washing him. There is no history of recurrent urinary tract infection, redness, soreness, or urinary retention. Which is the *single* most appropriate action? ★★

A Advise conservative management and provide reassurance

B Advise regular parental retraction

C Prescribe topical steroid

D Suggest circumcision

E Suggest surgical retraction and separation of adhesions

10. A 3-year-old boy with Down's syndrome is brought to the paediatric clinic by his mother, with constipation and intermittent offensive diarrhoea. He is in the lower quartile of weight for his age. A plain abdominal X-ray shows dilated colon to the level of a transition zone and contrast enema shows dilated colon but a less distensible rectum. Which is the *single* most appropriate next action? ★★

A Anorectal manometry

B Colonoscopy

C Flexible sigmoidoscopy

D Genetic counselling for the family

E Rectal mucosal suction biopsy

11. A child born prematurely at 38 weeks of gestation develops abdominal distension, vomiting, and diarrhoea with blood and mucus on the neonatal intensive care unit. A plain abdominal X-ray shows pneumatosis intestinalis and oedematous bowel, but no free gas. Which is the *single* most appropriate initial management? ★

A IV fluids and antibiotics

B IV fluids and bowel resection

C IV fluids and peritoneal drainage

D Place the child in isolation

E Total parenteral nutrition

12. A newborn baby with Down's syndrome has a 7cm mid-abdominal defect with an intact hernial sac containing bowel and viscera. Which is the *single* most appropriate next step in his management? ★★★

A Check the blood sugar

B Encourage epithelialization of the hernial sac with silver paste

C Obtain a plain abdominal radiograph

D Obtain cardiac imaging

E Undertake surgical reduction and primary closure of the defect

Extended Matching Questions

Paediatric urology

For each scenario choose the *single* most appropriate diagnosis from the list of options. Each option may be used once, more than once, or not at all.

A Epididymal cyst

B Epididymo-orchitis

C Femoral hernia

D Hydrocoele

E Inguinal hernia

F Nephroblastoma

G Obturator hernia

H Testicular torsion

I Testicular tumour

J Undescended testis

K Varicocoele

1. A 2-year-old boy has a smoothly enlarged scrotum surrounding normal testis. The scrotum transilluminates when a pen torch is applied. ★

2. A 13-year-old boy has developed tenderness in his testicle on the day of presentation to his GP. He has an absent ipsilateral cremasteric reflex. ★★

3. A 5-year-old boy has back pain and weight loss of about 0.5kg. He has a palpable mass in the left scrotum which feels like a mesh of dilated veins. ★★★

4. A 5-year-old boy has an intermittent, painless swelling in the inguinal canal. He has thickening of the spermatic cord. ★★

5. A 15-year-old boy develops a tender testicle, but normal cremasteric reflex, following a recent viral infection associated with painful facial swelling. ★★

Lumps in the neck

In a young patient with findings on examination as described choose the *single* most likely diagnosis from the list of options. Each option may be used once, more than once, or not at all.

A Branchial cyst

B Cystic hygroma

C Dermoid cyst

D Lymphadenopathy

E Parathyroid tumour

F Parotitis

G Pharyngeal pouch

H Sebaceous cyst

I Thyroglossal cyst

J Thyroid goitre

K Thyroid tumour

6. A transilluminable, painless midline cyst which moves on swallowing and tongue protrusion. ★★

7. Left-sided painless lump, lying at the anterior border at the junction of the middle and upper third of sternocleidomastoid muscle. ★★

8. Pea-sized lump on the back of the neck with a central punctum. ★

9. Midline mass, just above the hyoid bone, which does not move on tongue protrusion. ★★

10. Painless transilluminable lump in the posterior triangle of the neck. ★★★

ANSWERS

Single Best Answers

1. C ★★   OH Clin Surg, 4th edn → p428

The symptoms described are the key symptoms for making this diagnosis in the postnatal period. Nearly 30% of potentially lethal oesophageal abnormalities are associated with maternal polyhydramnios. Oesophageal atresia may be diagnosed on prenatal ultrasound scan. Classification of this condition is shown in Figure 11.2. Tracheo-oesophageal fistulas are present in the majority of cases, and are associated with cyanosis from aspiration upon feeding. Treatment of oesophageal atresia depends on the severity and will involve surgical repair to fix the fistula and reconnect the two ends of the oesophagus. Complex reconstruction may be required if the two ends are far apart. Postoperative complications include anastomotic leak, and later in life the child may be at risk of gastro-oesophageal reflux disease or even tracheomalacia. Pyloric stenosis presents at 3–8 weeks of age and is associated with projectile vomiting and not drooling. Duodenal atresia is associated with bile-stained vomiting as is annular pancreas, an embryological abnormality in which a portion of the pancreas remains wrapped around the duodenum. Pharyngeal pouches are classically acquired diverticula, typically affecting the elderly.

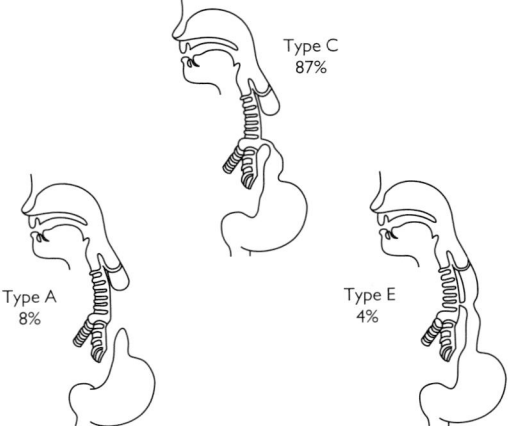

Figure 11.2 Maternal polyhydramnios
Reproduced from McLatchie et al., *Oxford Handbook of Clinical Surgery*, 4th edition, with permission from Oxford University Press.

2. C ★★★   OH Clin Surg, 4th edn → p432

The duplex ultrasound scan suggests that this child has a small bowel malrotation. A barium meal is not required as the diagnosis is not in doubt. After resuscitation with IV fluids and decompression of the stomach with a nasogastric tube, to reduce risk of aspiration under anaesthesia, exploratory laparotomy should be performed. Insertion of a nasogastric tube alone, without fluid resuscitation, combined with a 24h period of conservative management is inappropriate and risks extensive bowel infarction. Small bowel that has twisted on its mesenteric pedicle (resulting in ischaemia and necrosis) may require resection, however, in young children there is a significant risk of short bowel syndrome. If there are patchy ischaemic changes 'second look' laparotomy may be performed to review the bowel 24h later, before resection. A duplex scan may reveal poor blood flow to the small bowel and in this case has been used to distinguish superior mesenteric artery from superior mesenteric vein. Barium enema is not recommended since it is not as specific and sensitive as upper GI contrast study.

3. B ★★★   OH Clin Surg, 4th edn → pp424, 430

Neonatal physiology is very different to adolescent or adult physiology. They are not 'small adults'. It is essential to weigh a baby before starting treatment. Paediatric maintenance fluid should provide the glucose and electrolyte requirements. A neonate normally requires 2–3mmol/kg of potassium daily, but in hypokalaemia, as may occur with projectile vomiting, the baby may require more. Neonatal blood volume is 80mL/kg. Normal neonatal oral fluid intake should be approximately 150mL/kg/day. Neonatal blood pressure is low compared to adults and adolescents (40–50mmHg).

4. E ★★   OH Clin Surg, 4th edn → p430

Hypertrophic pyloric stenosis occurs four times more commonly in boys than girls and typically presents between 3 and 8 weeks of age. The baby is often eager to feed after vomiting. Loss of chloride and protons in vomit results in a hypochloraemic alkalosis. Some potassium is lost in vomit but the major cause of hypokalaemia is a result of renal loss secondary to the release of aldosterone in an attempt to correct dehydration hampered by low serum chloride. This drives the kidney to retain sodium and excrete potassium.

5. B ★★   OH Clin Surg, 4th edn → p435

Biliary atresia results in bilirubinaemia not bilious vomiting; both duodenal and jejuno-ileal obstruction, are distal enough to cause bilious vomiting. However, only duodenal atresia results in the 'double bubble' sign as no gas can pass distal to the duodenum. Pancreas divisum arises when the ventral and dorsal pancreatic ducts fail to fuse during embryological development. The main pancreatic duct drains via an accessory ampulla.

This can cause chronic pancreatitis although most patients remain asymptomatic. Pyloric stenosis is an obstruction too proximal to allow bilious vomiting.

6. C ★★ OH Clin Surg, 4th edn → p450

Undescended testicles are associated with a fourfold increase in risk of testicular cancer and also with delayed presentation of malignancy due to a lack of awareness of a testicular lump. Ninety-five per cent of retractile testicles descend into the scrotum spontaneously before puberty. Testicular agenesis is rare although apparent absence of testicles may occur as a result of secondary atrophy due to impaired blood supply in the perinatal period. An undescended testis occurs in approximately 2–4% of newborn boys, falling to 1.5% at 6 months. Undescended or incompletely descended testes rarely present with torsion. An undescended (as opposed to retractile) testicle should be brought to the scrotum at 1–2 years of age to avoid secondary damage due to trauma, torsion or increased ambient temperature. An intracanalicular or ectopic testicle can usually be managed by one-stage orchidopexy. Intra-abdominal testicles can be brought down with one- or two-stage orchidopexy with 50–90% success.

7. E ★★ OH Clin Surg, 4th edn → p434

This child is suffering from intussusception (see Figure 11.3). Air contrast enema is invasive and carries the risk of perforation and so is second choice to ultrasound for diagnosis. However it is the mainstay of treatment, being effective in 75% of cases. Occasionally diatrizoic acid (high-osmolality contrast agent) enema is required for diagnosis. Barium is never used, as it is hard to remove if it leaks through a perforation into the abdominal cavity. CT is avoided in this age group due to the radiation exposure and because general anaesthesia is usually required to ensure the child does not move during the investigation.

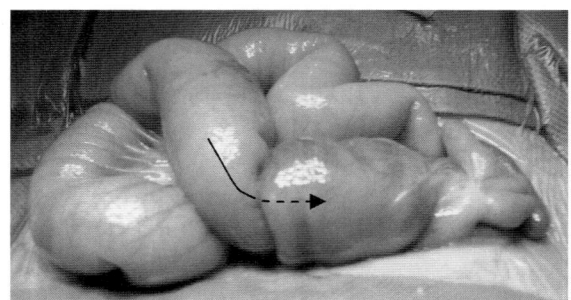

Figure 11.3 Intussusception
Reproduced from Gardiner and Borley, *Oxford Specialty Training in Surgery*, 2009, with permission from Oxford University Press.

8. B ★ OH Clin Surg, 4th edn → pp436, 438

This child is suffering from meconium ileus—abnormally thick meconium impacted within the lumen of normal bowel. This is pathognomonic of cystic fibrosis. See Figure 11.4. One of the presenting symptoms of Hirschsprung's disease may also be failure to pass meconium, but 'bright spots', due to the echogenicity of meconium on antenatal ultrasound scan, are associated with cystic fibrosis. Anorectal malformation would present with distal obstruction and absence of, or an abnormally sited anus, is usually recognized at the neonatal check. Jejuno-ileal atresia or an obstructing small bowel malrotation are more proximal small bowel obstructions that do not obstruct the passage of meconium.

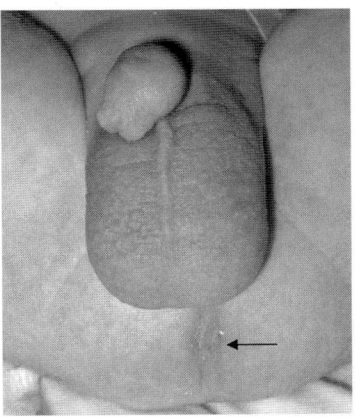

Figure 11.4 Imperforate anus
Reproduced from Gardiner and Borley, *Oxford Specialty Training in Surgery*, 2009, with permission from Oxford University Press.

9. A ★★ OH Clin Surg, 4th edn → p448

This is the most common referral seen in paediatric surgery. Remember that the prepuce (foreskin) is fused to the penile glans at birth and gradually separates (10% of 5-year-olds will have a non-retractable foreskin). Only if symptomatic should treatment be offered—initially bathing and gentle retraction; topical 1% hydrocortisone may speed separation of adhesions and relieves symptoms of inflammation, but would not be the initial choice of treatment here. Antibiotics may be given if balanitis is present (see Figure 11.5). Preputioplasty (retraction under anaesthetic) and circumcision are offered to boys with a phimosis (a non-retractable foreskin) associated with scarring, often due to balanitis xerotica obliterans, that will not resolve.

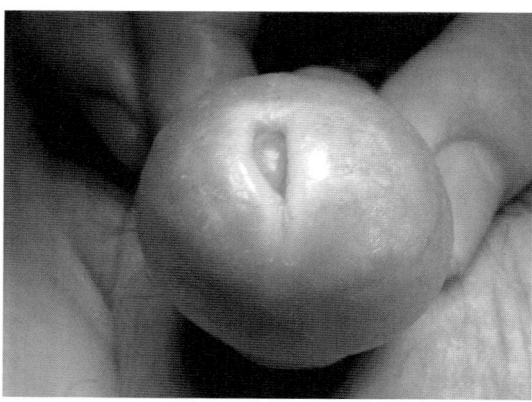

Figure 11.5 Balanitis
Reproduced from Gardiner and Borley, *Oxford Specialty Training in Surgery*, 2009, with permission from Oxford University Press.

10. E ★★   OH Clin Surg, 4th edn → p436

Rectal biopsy is likely to show aganglionosis, caused by failure of migration of neural crest cells into the hindgut, diagnostic of Hirschsprung's disease. Genetic counselling is not indicated as the diagnosis of Down's syndrome has been established. Both colonoscopy and flexible sigmoidoscopy are relatively invasive. Anorectal manometry is reserved for older children with later presentations of lower bowel disturbances who will tolerate this investigation, and may demonstrate failure of anal relaxation on rectal balloon distension due to loss of the recto-anal inhibitory reflex.

11. A ★   OH Clin Surg, 4th edn → p442

Necrotizing enterocolitis is associated with premature delivery, formula milk feeds, hypoxia, and systemic sepsis. It is associated with 'micro-epidemics' in neonatal wards but additional isolation measures are not required. Treatment is directed to dealing with complications. Fluid resuscitation and antibiotics, total parenteral nutrition, and bowel rest are the initial steps, in that order. Surgery is the next step for advanced disease with perforation or intestinal ischaemia—initially peritoneal drainage and then resection if there is bowel necrosis. Neonatal mortality from perforated necrotizing enterocolitis is 40%.

→ Morgan J, Young L, McGuire W. Slow advancement of enteral feed volumes to prevent necrotizing enterocolitis in very low birth weight infants. *Cochrane Database Syst Rev* 2011; (3):CD001241.

12. A ★★★ OH Clin Surg, 4th edn → p440

Exomphalos is associated with many genetic/developmental defects that also cause renal and cardiac anomalies. The condition is associated with hyperinsulinaemia, and so blood sugar should be checked initially, as part of early resuscitation, allowing correction of hypoglycaemia. Newborn babies with this condition should subsequently have cardiac imaging prior to further management. Assessment of lung hypoplasia must also be undertaken. If the condition is detected by antenatal ultrasound scan, caesarean section is likely to be performed. Exomphalos minor (defect <5cm, only bowel herniated) may be treated with primary closure. Exomphalos major (defect >5cm, herniated bowel and viscera—see Figure 11.6) is usually treated by encouraging epithelialization until the abdominal cavity has matured enough to have capacity to allow hernia reduction. Plain abdominal radiograph is not likely to be helpful at this point unless there are signs of obstruction. The key is to protect the hernial sac and thus the abdominal organs whilst investigations are performed.

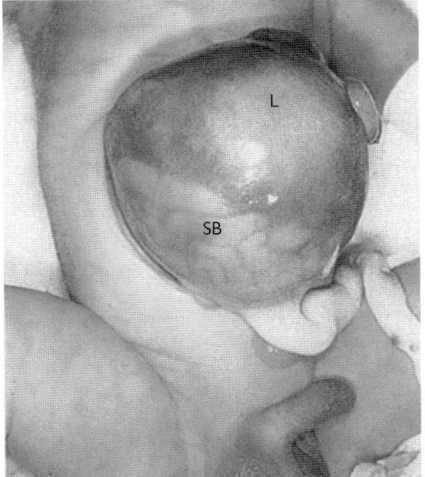

Figure 11.6 Exomphalos major
Reproduced from Morris and Wood, *Oxford Textbook of Surgery*, 2nd edition, 2000, with permission from Oxford University Press.

Extended Matching Questions

1. D ★

Classical presentation of hydrocoele.

2. H ★★

Testicular torsion—the usual presentation is one of an acutely tender testis, lying high and transversely in the scrotum associated with an absent cremasteric reflex.

3. K ★★★

The initial presentation is suspicious of varicocoele. However, left-sided disease and a history of back pain and weight loss, raises the possibility of a renal tumour compressing or invading the left renal vein.

4. E ★★

A good history for inguinal hernia and often cord thickening is the only finding in children at examination.

5. B ★★

Epididymo-orchitis is the likely diagnosis although high index of suspicion for torsion should be maintained. Orchitis is the most common complication of mumps in post-pubertal men, affecting about 20–30% of cases. Orchitis usually occurs 1–2 weeks after parotitis. Of affected testicles, 30–50% show a degree of testicular atrophy.

→ Masarani M, Wazait H, Dinneen H. Mumps orchitis. *J R Soc Med* 2006; 99(11):573–5.

6. I ★★

Thyroglossal cysts usually occur at or below the level of the hyoid bone and rise with tongue protrusion. They are fluid-filled structures arising from incomplete closure of the thyroglossal duct. They may become infected or form a sinus. In this case they are best excised along with any remnants of the thyroglossal tract.

7. A ★★

A branchial cyst most commonly presents in young adults as a smooth swelling. Fluid aspirate may contain cholesterol crystals visible on microscopy. Infection may result in development of a branchial abscess.

8. H ★

Sebaceous cysts, or epidermoid cysts, although not common in children can occur anywhere, but scalp and back of neck are more frequent locations. The small punctum denotes the epidermal origin, which has the potential to become infected and cause abscess formation.

9. C ★★

A dermoid cyst is a developmental inclusion cyst. They are commonly found at the upper lateral margin of the orbit.

10. B ★★★

This is the typical position for a cystic hygroma, a benign, multiloculated embryological malformation of the lymphatics. Seventy-five per cent arise in the neck.

These are often large, poorly circumscribed lesions which may cause stridor in the neonate or in early infancy. They may be extensive, occurring in the axilla, or extending from the neck into the mediastinum or chest, requiring CT or MRI to determine relationship with other structures. Surgical excision may be required although sclerotherapy is an alternative. Ten per cent recur.

Chapter 12

Trauma surgery

Sebastian Dawson-Bowling and Serena Ledwidge

Appreciation of the 'golden hour' for resuscitation, and adoption of principles of the advanced trauma life support (ATLS) system are key factors in improving outcome for the patient with major injuries. Adherence to the strict protocols of the ABCDEs of the primary survey enables the trauma team to identify and deal with life-threatening conditions, prior to definitive treatment of problems with lesser immediacy.

The clinician who understands the mechanism of injury will maintain heightened levels of suspicion for clinical signs which point to well-recognized conditions resulting in early mortality and morbidity, for instance, tension pneumothorax, cardiac tamponade, and rising intracranial pressure.

This chapter will probe your grasp of the principles of trauma management. You will also be tested on common patterns of thoracic, abdominal, vascular, and cranial injuries.

Whilst clinical presentations of civilian trauma have remained consistent in recent years, the impact of military trauma in worldwide theatres of conflict has stimulated numerous advances in the management of trauma. The current impetus for reorganization of trauma services in the UK is tacit acknowledgement of the improvement in outcomes that can be achieved by adherence to recognized protocols in this challenging and demanding field of surgery.

Frank Smith

QUESTIONS

Single Best Answers

1. A 27-year-old motorcyclist is involved in a high speed collision with an oncoming car and is thrown 20 metres. The ambulance team immobilize his cervical spine. On arrival in the emergency department, he is alert. Heart rate is 130bpm and blood pressure 70/40mmHg. His trachea is deviated to the left, his right hemithorax is hyperresonant to percussion, and his respiratory rate is 42 breaths per minute. He is speaking in single-word sentences. Which is the *single* most appropriate next step in his management? ★

A Insert 12G cannula into right 2nd intercostal space, mid-clavicular line

B Insert right-sided chest drain via 5th intercostal space, between the anterior and mid-axillary lines

C Obtain urgent portable chest X-ray to clarify diagnosis

D Protect airway with immediate endotracheal intubation

E Urgent infusion of crystalloid via two wide-bore IV cannulae

2. A 52-year-old man falls 1.5 metres from a ladder and sustains an injury to the side of his head. On arrival in hospital he is able to give a clear account of the events leading to his fall, but when reassessed 15min later his Glasgow Coma Scale (GCS) score has fallen to 8. Which is the *single* most likely reason for this? ★★

A Base of skull fracture with associated cerebrospinal fluid leak

B Extradural haemorrhage

C Hypovolaemic shock resulting in poor cerebral perfusion

D Neurogenic shock resulting in poor cerebral perfusion

E Subarachnoid haemorrhage

3. A 72-year-old man falls down a flight of stairs and sustains a severe head injury. When he arrives in hospital his GCS score is 10 and there is blood at the left external auditory meatus. Which is the *single* most appropriate first management? ★★

A Assess the patient's airway and immobilize the cervical spine

B Document the GCS to allow serial neurological observations

C Obtain an urgent CT scan of the head

D Obtain collateral history regarding the use of alcohol or drugs which may confuse the clinical picture

E Obtain portable radiographs of the neck to exclude concurrent cervical spine injury

4. A 40-year-old woman arrives in the emergency department having been stabbed in the upper left quadrant of her abdomen. She is confused but conscious, and there are no other injuries. After rapid administration of 2L of crystalloid followed by 2 units of O-negative blood, her blood pressure is 65/30mmHg and heart rate is 160bpm. Which is the *single* most appropriate next step in her management? ★★★

A Admit to ward for serial abdominal examinations to assess for developing peritonism

B Arrange urgent abdominal CT to assess for visceral injury

C Cross-match 6 units of packed red cells and assess haemodynamic response to further rapid blood transfusion

D Perform diagnostic peritoneal lavage in emergency department

E Transfer to operating theatre for immediate laparotomy

5. A 32-year-old cyclist is hit by a van at high speed. In the ambulance she is intubated and her cervical spine immobilized. Two litres of crystalloid and 2 units of O-negative blood are administered. On arrival in the emergency department her heart rate is 140bpm, blood pressure is 85/59mmHg, and she has distended neck veins. Auscultation of her chest reveals equal air entry bilaterally but faint heart sounds. Which is the *single* most appropriate next step in her management? ★★★

A Emergency pericardiocentesis via insertion of cannula 2cm inferior to xiphochondral junction

B Immediate needle chest decompression via 2nd intercostal space, mid-clavicular line

C Insert large bore, left-sided chest-drain via 5th intercostal space anterior and mid-axillary line

D Obtain chest X-ray to assess for possible rib fractures and associated pneumothorax

E Urgent CT scan of chest, abdomen, and pelvis to assess all possible bleeding sites

6. An 8-year-old girl falls off a trampoline sustaining an open fracture to her left tibia and fibula. In the emergency department the wound is covered and the limb is splinted. Opioid analgesia is administered and she is transferred to the ward for elevation of the limb. An hour later, despite further opioid analgesia, she is screaming in pain. Her pain is exacerbated by passive dorsiflexion of the left foot, and persists after removal of the splint and elevation. Capillary refill in the left foot is delayed but her dorsalis pedis and posterior tibial pulses remain palpable. Which is the *single* most appropriate treatment at this stage? ★

A Administer Entonox and further opioid analgesia

B Apply a well moulded plaster-cast in an attempt to optimize reduction of the fracture

C Arrange urgent arteriogram to assess for occult arterial injury

D Arrange urgent transfer to theatre for emergency fasciotomy

E Initiate immediate streptokinase infusion to break down potential arterial thrombus

7. A 53-year-old woman falls down 15 stairs sustaining an open fracture of her right femur and several broken ribs. On arrival in the emergency department she is alert but anxious. Her heart rate is 110bpm, blood pressure is 120/102mmHg, and respiratory rate is 28 breaths per minute. Which is the *single* most accurate estimation of her current blood loss? ★★★★

A 250mL

B 1200mL

C 2.0L

D 2.5L

E 3.5L

8. A 45-year-old factory worker is caught under a forklift truck as it reverses. On arrival in hospital his blood pressure is 78/54mmHg, heart rate is 135bpm, and he shows no haemodynamic response to the administration of 2L of Hartmann's solution and 2 units of blood. There is no clinical evidence of a chest injury, but he has significant bruising in the suprapubic region and blood at the urethral meatus. Although not deformed, the right leg appears slightly shorter than the left. Which is the *single* most important next step in his management? ★★★★

A Compression of pelvic ring using bedsheet

B Contact general surgeons for consideration of urgent laparotomy

C Transfer to radiology department for arterial embolization

D Transfer to theatre for open reduction and internal fixation of pelvis

E Urgent CT scan of chest, abdomen, and pelvis to assess all possible bleeding sites

9. A 72-year-old woman falls down a flight of 11 stairs in her house and attends the emergency department with pain and tenderness in her neck. Her cervical spine is triple immobilized on admission using a collar and blocks. She is haemodynamically stable and has oxygen saturation levels of 99% on room air. She has no neurological deficit. A C-spine radiograph is obtained (see Figure 12.1). A radiographer's report accompanies the image and states 'no fracture visualized on this image'.

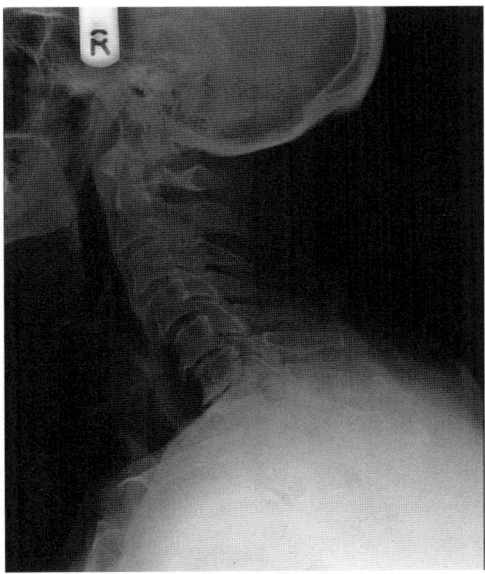

Figure 12.1 The C-spine radiograph

Which is the *single* most appropriate next step in her management? ★★

A Facet joint injections to reduce inflammation around cervical vertebrae

B High-dose methylprednisolone therapy

C Reassure and discharge home with simple analgesia

D Soft collar and admit for serial neurological observations

E Urgent CT scan

10. A car is involved in a high-speed collision with an oncoming lorry. The passenger, a 53-year-old female, is ejected from the vehicle. On arrival in the emergency department she is haemodynamically stable and breathing normally. However, there is pain, bruising, and tenderness in her back and she has no movement in either lower limb. Sensation is normal at the level of the umbilicus, reduced between the umbilicus and the pubic symphysis, and completely absent distal to this. Which is the *single* most accurate description of her spinal level? ★★★★

A T10

B T11

C T12

D L1

E L2

11. A 37-year-old motorcyclist crashes at high speed. On arrival in hospital his cervical spine is immobilized and his airway and breathing optimized. After initial fluid resuscitation with 2L of Hartmann's solution he remains hypotensive and tachycardic. His right femur is deformed, and he has continued pulsatile bleeding from a wound in the middle of the right thigh. Which is the *single* most appropriate next step in his management? ★★

A Apply temporary splint to right thigh whilst applying direct pressure over bleeding point

B Apply tourniquet to thigh proximal to injury whilst continuing further Hartmann's infusion

C Obtain radiographs of both right femur and right tibia to exclude possible sequential lower limb fractures

D Obtain radiographs of right femur to assess severity of fracture

E Undertake blunt dissection to identify bleeding vessel and allow application of arterial clamp

12. A 22-year-old medical student falls from a balcony at a party sustaining an injury to his right chest wall. On arrival in the emergency department he is confused and speaking in single-word sentences. His respiratory rate is 25 breaths per minute and oxygen saturation 89% on air. His right hemithorax is hyperresonant, there is a 3 × 2cm wound lateral to the right nipple, and the trachea is central. Which is the *single* most appropriate first step in his management? ★★★★

A Chest needle decompression via 2nd intercostal space, mid-clavicular line

B Immediate endotracheal intubation

C Insertion of chest drain via the chest wound

D Sterile occlusive dressing taped down on three sides

E Urgent CT scan of chest to exclude pericardial injury

13. A major incident is called in the emergency department after an explosion in a factory. Five men are injured and all require catheterization as part of their management. In which *single* patient may urethral catheterization be considered? ★★★

A Blood at the urethral meatus

B High riding prostate on rectal examination

C Inability to micturate

D Penetrating injury to suprapubic region

E Scrotal haematoma

14. A 27-year-old woman is a passenger in a car crash at 80 miles per hour and sustains multiple injuries to her chest, limbs, and cervical spine. A large right pneumothorax is identified and a chest drain inserted. Following transfer to intensive care for monitoring, she is found to have persistent profuse bubbling through the underwater seal of her chest drain. Which is the *single* most likely explanation for this? ★★★★

A Gastric rupture

B Incorrect connection of chest drainage system

C Missed contralateral pneumothorax

D Oesophageal rupture

E Tracheobronchial rupture

Extended Matching Questions

Emergency interventions

For each scenario choose the *single* most appropriate next intervention from the list of options. Each option may be used once, more than once, or not at all.

A Chest drain insertion

B Discharge home for GP follow-up

C Emergency chest decompression with cannula

D Emergency thoracotomy

E Endotracheal intubation

F Nasogastric tube insertion

G Needle pericardiocentesis

H Surgical cricothyroidotomy

I Urgent bronchoscopy

1. An 80-year-old man is brought to the emergency department having been found lying at the bottom of the stairs in his nursing home. On arrival in hospital his GCS score is 8. Air entry is equal throughout all lung zones but his breathing is noisy and his oxygen saturation on air is 88%. ★★★★

2. A 32-year-old woman is rescued by firefighters from the second storey of a burning building. On arrival she is found to have burns to her face and right arm, with singeing of her eyebrows. She is coughing up black sputum, her voice is hoarse, and stridor is audible. ★★★

3. A 50-year-old man is assaulted and sustains injuries to his face and neck. On arrival in hospital his neck is swollen and he is in significant respiratory distress, although managing the odd word in a hoarse voice. The vocal cords cannot be visualized with a laryngoscope. ★★★

4. A 19-year-old nursing student is knocked from her bicycle by a car travelling at 15 miles per hour and strikes her left chest wall against the handlebars as she falls. In the emergency department a chest X-ray shows simple fracture to the 5th and 6th ribs and a moderate sized pneumothorax. Her respiratory rate is 28/min and oxygen saturation on room air is 93%. ★

5. A 36-year-old policeman is assaulted and sustains an isolated heavy blow to the right chest wall with a baseball bat. His SaO_2 on 15L of oxygen is 83%, and part of his chest wall is seen to be moving inwards during expiration, outwards during expiration. His chest X-ray shows comminuted fractures of the 3rd, 4th, and 5th ribs but no obvious pneumothorax. ★★★★

Diagnosis of traumatic injury

For each scenario choose the *single* most likely diagnosis from the list of options. Each option may be used once, more than once, or not at all.

A Aortic rupture

B Cardiac tamponade

C Diaphragmatic rupture

D Flail chest

E Haemothorax

F Oesophageal rupture

G Pneumothorax

H Pulmonary contusion

I Tension pneumothorax

6. A 23-year-old man driving a car hits the back of a lorry at 50 miles per hour. His chest strikes the steering wheel. A chest radiograph obtained during primary survey shows widening of the mediastinum. Five minutes later the patient sustains a cardiopulmonary arrest. ★★★

7. A 5-year-old boy loses control of his bike on a hill and crashes into a fence. He is thrown against the handlebars at speed sustaining a blow to his chest. On initial assessment in the emergency department he is haemodynamically stable with oxygen saturation of 92% on air; 40min later this has fallen to 88% on air. His chest X-ray shows no abnormality. ★★★★

8. A 32-year-old man is stabbed in the right side of the chest. Following initial fluid resuscitation in the ambulance his blood pressure is 92/69mmHg and pulse 120bpm. Dullness to percussion is found in the right lower and mid-zones, and right chest air entry is reduced. ★

9. A 72-year-old woman falls down three steps sustaining a blow to her right chest wall subsequent to which she develops immediate pain in her lower ribs. Examination reveals hyperresonance to percussion with reduced right-sided air entry. The trachea is central and she remains haemodynamically stable. ★

10. A 54 year old man riding a motorcycle is brought to hospital after crashing into a lamp-post and sustaining a direct blow to his sternum. Chest X-ray shows no evidence of bony injury, but a left-sided haemopneumothorax is present. A chest drain is inserted and the blood in the tube is seen to contain particulate matter. ★★★

Head trauma

For each scenario choose the *single* most appropriate next intervention from the list of options. Each option may be used once, more than once, or not at all.

A Administer high-dose IV methylprednisolone

B Admit for overnight neurological observations

C Discharge home with head injury advice sheet

D Discussion with relatives regarding withdrawal of treatment and possible organ donation

E Obtain urgent head CT scan

F Refer to nearest neurosurgical unit for urgent bone flap craniotomy

G Temperature normalization with blankets and warm peritoneal lavage followed by neurological re-evaluation

H Through lavage and wound closure under local anaesthesia

I Undertake immediate burr-hole cranial decompression under sterile conditions in emergency department

11. A 16-year-old girl loses control of her toboggan and hits a tree at speed, sustaining a significant head injury. She is discovered several hours later lying unconscious in the snow, and in the emergency department she has a GCS score of 3, doll's eye reflexes with non-reactive pupils, absent gag and corneal reflexes, and a core temperature of 30°C. She is making no spontaneous ventilatory effort. ★★★

12. A 48-year-old man is assaulted with a wooden plank and sustains a single blow to the head. Two hours following arrival in hospital he has a GCS score of 14 and there is no other evidence of neurological injury. A CT scan of his head shows a skull fracture with a 4mm depression, and there is a bleeding laceration of the overlying skin. ★★★★

13. A 40-year-old man who lives alone trips coming out of the pub and knocks his head. Although he briefly loses consciousness at the scene, his GCS score on arrival in hospital is 14, and 2h later this has risen to 15. He smells strongly of alcohol. ★★

14. An 80-year-old woman trips in her porch and strikes her head against the stone steps as she falls. In the emergency department her GCS score is found to be falling steadily, and CT scan demonstrates a large right-sided extradural haematoma. ★★★

15. A 52-year-old cyclist is knocked over by a slow-moving van, sustaining an isolated head injury and losing consciousness for 4min. There is one episode of vomiting in the ambulance and GCS score on arrival in the emergency department is 13. An hour later her GCS score is 15 and there is no focal neurology. ★★

Abdominal trauma

For each scenario choose the *single* most appropriate next intervention from the list of options. Each option may be used once, more than once, or not at all.

A Admission for close observation and serial clinical reassessment
B Diagnostic peritoneal lavage
C Discharge with abdominal injury advice sheet
D Endotracheal intubation
E Immediate MRI of abdomen and pelvis
F Nasogastric tube insertion
G Transfer to facility with surgical capabilities on site
H Transfer to theatre for emergency laparotomy
I Urgent laparoscopy

16. A 30-year old man is assaulted on his way home from work, sustaining repeated stab injuries to the neck, chest, and abdomen. Primary survey reveals blood pressure of 75/48mmHg, heart rate of 136bpm, and SaO$_2$ on 15L of oxygen is 83%. Active bleeding is visible from both his chest and abdomen. There is copious blood in his larynx and pharynx and gurgling sounds are audible as he breathes. ★

17. A 52-year-old woman is brought to the emergency department following the accidental discharge of a rifle at medium range, as a result of which she has sustained an isolated bullet wound to her abdomen. An entry point but no exit wound is visible. After initial fluid resuscitation her heart rate is 103bpm and blood pressure 105/65mmHg. ★★★

18. A 53-year-old man loses control of his car at 40 miles per hour and veers into a wall. The airbag fails to deploy and he is struck in the abdomen by the steering wheel. In hospital his blood pressure is 95/78mmHg and heart rate is 98bpm. Erect chest X-ray shows air under the right hemidiaphragm. ★★★

19. A 37-year-old motorcyclist crashes into the central reservation of a dual carriageway and the barrier strikes him in the abdomen. No other injuries are identified. CT scan reveals a 3cm laceration to the left lobe of the liver. Following initial fluid resuscitation in the emergency department his blood pressure is 110/78mmHg and heart rate is 92bpm. ★★★

20. A 60-year-old man walking his dog in the park is attacked and stabbed in the back. He presents to his local cottage hospital with a 3cm knife-wound to the right of his L3 vertebra. Urinalysis shows a small number of red cells but he is haemodynamically stable throughout. ★★★

ANSWERS

Single Best Answers

1. A ★   OH Clin Surg, 4th edn → p480

This patient has a tension pneumothorax, a medical emergency requiring immediate treatment on clinical grounds alone. Management should never be delayed to obtain imaging. Immediate chest decompression via a cannula should be followed by definitive siting of a chest drain, but chest drain insertion takes time and should not be the first line of treatment. The patient is speaking, ruling out significant airway compromise. Although haemodynamic compromise should be suspected in all trauma patients, circulatory issues should not be addressed until the patient's breathing has been appropriately stabilized.

→ http://www.facs.org/trauma/atls

2. B ★★   OH Clin Surg, 4th edn → p486

This is the classic 'talk-and-die' presentation of an extradural haemorrhage, characterized by the presence of a lucid interval, before build-up of blood causes loss of consciousness. Urgent neurosurgical referral is mandatory. The commonest cause is injury to the middle meningeal artery, deep to the temporal bone.

Base of skull fracture often causes cerebrospinal fluid leakage but in isolation is unlikely to cause rapid loss of consciousness. Subarachnoid haemorrhage does not usually occur as a result of head injury. It is unlikely that either hypovolaemic or neurogenic shock would manifest as a delayed loss of consciousness, although the management of all trauma patients must include a detailed circulatory assessment.

3. A ★★   OH Clin Surg, 4th edn → p478

All trauma patients should be managed according to the ATLS system of 'ABCDE'. The assessment and securing of an airway, with concomitant C-spine immobilization, are followed by optimization of breathing and circulation—without these, the risk of further 'secondary' brain injury from hypoxia or hypoperfusion is high. Only once the patient's respiratory and circulatory status have been optimized should 'D' (disability) be addressed. Exposure follows and requires a complete 'top to toe' examination. In practice, different members of the trauma team may deal with different parts of the algorithm simultaneously, but this order outlines how to prioritize systems.

→ http://www.facs.org/trauma/atls

4. E ★★★   OH Clin Surg, 4th edn → p482

Sharp abdominal injury with haemodynamic instability is an absolute indication for emergency laparotomy. This patient's failure to demonstrate any haemodynamic response to fluid resuscitation measures results from continued intra-abdominal bleeding, probably due to splenic injury. Immediate surgical control of the bleeding source must be achieved. Further clinical assessment, investigation (such as a focused assessment with sonography for trauma (FAST) scan or diagnostic peritoneal lavage) or attempts at fluid challenge will only delay definitive treatment and are therefore contraindicated.

→ http://www.facs.org/trauma/atls

5. A ★★★ OH Clin Surg, 4th edn → p486

Cardiac tamponade can result from either sharp or blunt trauma, and is classically characterized by Beck's triad of raised central venous pressure, tachycardia, and muffled heart sounds. Although pericardiocentesis is not definitive treatment it can be of considerable therapeutic benefit in the haemodynamically unstable patient. The diagnosis is clinical (although can be confirmed by echocardiography or ultrasonography), and treatment should not be delayed to obtain X-rays or CT scans. In the absence of clinical evidence of injury to the pleural cavity, there is no indication for either chest drain or needle chest decompression.

→ http://www.facs.org/trauma/atls

6. D ★ OH Clin Surg, 4th edn → p485

Compartment syndrome is a relatively common sequela of lower limb fractures, and is characterized by pain out of proportion to the injury, exacerbated by passive stretching of the muscles within the affected compartment. Common pitfalls are to assume that compartment syndrome cannot occur with open fractures, or that it is excluded by the presence of distal pulses. Absent pulses are late features suggesting likely irreversible soft tissue damage.

In the awake patient diagnosis should be made on clinical grounds alone, and emergency surgical decompression should not be delayed for further investigation.

→ http://www.facs.org/trauma/atls

7. B ★★★★ OH Clin Surg, 4th edn → p479

Haemorrhage is conventionally classified into four classes based on percentage of total volume lost. Although exact quantification is clearly difficult in the acute setting, estimation is helpful in gauging initial fluid requirements. For a patient weighing 70kg, with circulating volume of approximately 5L, the classification is shown in Table 12.1 (a useful aide-mémoire is to think of tennis scores).

Patients in class I–II shock may initially be resuscitated with 2L of warmed crystalloid. Class III–IV shock is an indication for 2L crystalloid immediately followed with 2 units of blood.

→ http://www.facs.org/trauma/atls

Table 12.1 Classification of haemorrhage

Class	Blood loss	Heart rate	Blood pressure	Respiratory rate	Conscious level
I	<15% (750mL)	<100	Normal	<20	Mildly anxious
II	15-30% (750–1500mL)	100–120	Normal systolic, raised diastolic	20–30	Anxious
III	30-40% (1500–2000mL)	120–140	Reduced	30–40	Confused
IV	>40% (2000mL)	>140	Reduced	40	Drowsy

8. A ★★★★   OH Clin Surg, 4th edn → pp482–3

The apparent urethral injury, pelvic/lower limb asymmetry, and bruising suggest a pelvic fracture; the presence of haemodynamic instability indicates possible disruption of intrapelvic vessels (more commonly veins). In many cases, gentle splintage of the pelvis (either with a sheet or purpose-designed strap) will provide sufficient tamponade to control the bleeding. If not, either embolization or laparotomy may become necessary. If surgical stabilization is required to facilitate this, it can be undertaken temporarily with external fixation; definitive fracture fixation can be undertaken at a later stage. The unstable patient should not be transferred to the CT scanner.

→ http://www.facs.org/trauma/atls

9. E ★★   OH Clin Surg, 4th edn → p550

Review of C-spine radiographs in the trauma setting should ideally be undertaken by someone experienced in their interpretation. However, all doctors should have at their disposal a basic approach to assessing them. The radiographer's report is technically correct—no fractures are visible on this investigation. However, the first point is to check the adequacy of the lateral radiograph. This should extend distally as far as the C7–T1 junction; if it does not, the plain film should be repeated or a CT obtained. Until complete imaging is available, the C-spine cannot be cleared and full immobilization should remain. Although this lady's radiograph shows evidence of degenerative change, there is never any indication in the acute trauma setting for the use of either systemic steroids or facet joint injections.

→ http://www.facs.org/trauma/atls

10. A ★★★★   OH Clin Surg, 4th edn → p554

The spinal level is defined as the most caudal level at which both sensory and motor function are completely normal. The sensory level is the most caudal level at which sensation is completely normal; sensation at the level of the umbilicus is innervated by T10 (T12 at the symphysis pubis). Motor function at this level cannot be formally assessed as there is no skeletal muscle innervation between T2 and L1.

→ http://www.facs.org/trauma/atls

11. A ★★   OH Clin Surg, 4th edn → p538

This patient has an open femoral fracture with ongoing bleeding, causing persistent hypovolaemia despite initial fluid resuscitation. After 2L of crystalloid it would be appropriate to consider a blood transfusion. Control of bleeding in this situation is often best achieved by an approximate reduction and splintage of the fracture, accompanied by direct pressure over the bleeding point. Only in the presence of massive uncontrollable haemorrhage should a tourniquet be temporarily considered, and there is seldom a role for attempting to identify and clamp vessels in the emergency department. Obtaining X-rays at this stage would add nothing to the stabilization of the patient's haemodynamic status.

→ http://www.facs.org/trauma/atls

12. D ★★★★   OH Clin Surg, 4th edn → p480

An open pneumothorax, whilst not as immediately life-threatening as a tension pneumothorax, is nevertheless potentially fatal if left untreated. As the chest wall expands during inspiration, air preferentially enters the chest via the wound rather than the trachea, causing the pleural cavity to fill with air and deflate the lung. A dressing taped down on three sides will act as a 'flutter-valve', allowing air out but not in, thus re-inflating the lung. This should be promptly followed with chest drain placement at a site far from the open chest wound. Initial management should not be delayed to obtain CT or other detailed imaging.

→ http://www.facs.org/trauma/atls

13. D ★★★   OH Clin Surg, 4th edn → p533

Passage of a urethral catheter is routinely undertaken during the early assessment and management of the polytrauma patient to allow careful monitoring of fluid balance and renal perfusion, as well as bladder decompression. However, in the presence of any features suggestive of urethral injury, including difficulty in micturition, this should be delayed until a retrograde urethrogram is obtained; suprapubic catheterization may be necessary as an alternative. Sharp injury to the suprapubic region is highly unlikely to injure the urethra which lies entirely within the pelvis.

→ http://www.facs.org/trauma/atls

14. E ★★★★   OH Clin Surg, 4th edn → p480

Injury to the tracheobronchial tree is often associated with other non-survivable injuries. However, in patients who survive it should always be suspected when there is a persistent large air leak after chest drain insertion. Oesophageal injury may present with pneumothorax, but is much less likely to cause a persistent air leak. Air from a contralateral pneumothorax would not cross the mediastinum, and that from a gastric injury would be likely to remain under the diaphragm unless associated with a diaphragmatic injury. Incorrect drain connection is likely to lead to absent, rather than excessive bubbling of the drain.

→ http://www.facs.org/trauma/atls

Extended Matching Questions

1. E ★★★★ OH Clin Surg, 4th edn → pp486–7

This patient has clinical evidence of a significant head injury, as a result of which he is unconscious and unable to maintain his airway adequately. Endotracheal intubation should be performed at an early stage to prevent secondary hypoxic brain injury.

2. E ★★★ OH Clin Surg, 4th edn → pp604–6

Any patient sustaining burns should be assessed for concomitant inhalation injury, which can cause rapidly progressive upper airway narrowing. Facial burns, hoarseness, carbonaceous sputum, and singeing of facial hair all indicate potential inhalation injury, and if identified the threshold for endotracheal intubation should be low. Accompanying stridor virtually mandates intubation.

3. H ★★★ OH Clin Surg, 4th edn → p478

Maxillofacial trauma poses a high risk of airway compromise, especially if accompanied by head injury. As with all trauma patients, the first stage in the primary survey is to establish an adequate airway; if the vocal cords cannot be visualized a surgical airway may be the only available means. Significant neck swelling following neck trauma frequently indicates laryngeal fracture, in which case surgical cricothyroidotomy may be preferable to tracheostomy as an acute life-saving measure.

4. A ★ OH Clin Surg, 4th edn → pp480–1

An asymptomatic simple pneumothorax can be managed expectantly with close observation. However, this patient is moderately hypoxic and tachypnoeic; any sign of respiratory compromise indicates chest drain insertion with an underwater seal. Needle decompression may be appropriate if there is more profound respiratory distress but will only delay insertion of the chest drain in this case.

5. E ★★★★ OH Clin Surg, 4th edn → pp480–1

A flail chest is defined as two or more ribs fractured in two or more places; this causes paradoxical movement of the flail segment out of phase with the rest of the chest wall. The force to the thoracic wall required to produce such an injury frequently causes significant contusion damage to the underlying lung, often with severe respiratory compromise. Management is supportive, and a short period of intubation with positive pressure ventilation is often required to maintain adequate oxygenation.

→ http://www.facs.org/trauma/atls

6. A ★★★   OH Clin Surg, 4th edn → pp484–5

Aortic rupture is characteristically associated with rapid deceleration, and radiological features include mediastinal widening, right-sided oesophageal deviation, and obliteration of both the aortopulmonary window and aortic knob. The injury is often fatal at the scene; if not this is likely to be due to containment of haematoma by either clot or adventitia, and subsequent displacement of this leads to rapid exsanguination into the chest and is usually fatal. Patients with suspected aortic rupture therefore require immediate cardiothoracic referral.

7. H ★★★★   OH Clin Surg, 4th edn → pp480–1

In adults, pulmonary contusion is almost invariably accompanied by rib fractures, often with a flail chest segment. However, children's skeletons have a far greater degree of elasticity, such that significant lung injury often results from blunt chest trauma in the absence of rib or sternal fractures. This should be suspected in the presence of progressive hypoxia; intubation may become necessary.

8. E ★   OH Clin Surg, 4th edn → pp480–1

The combination of dullness to percussion and reduced air entry indicates fluid in the pleural cavity. In the presence of significant hypovolaemia following penetrating chest trauma this is due to a large haemothorax, and requires urgent fluid resuscitation and chest drain insertion, followed by cardiothoracic surgical intervention if the bleeding remains uncontrolled.

9. G ★   OH Clin Surg, 4th edn → pp480–1

Pneumothorax may result from rib fractures if sharp bone fragments penetrate the pleura and lung parenchyma, and may require chest drain insertion. A central trachea is useful in excluding a tension pneumothorax, although it should be remembered that a simple pneumothorax may progress to a tension pneumothorax. Adequate analgesia is essential as the reduced air entry and accompanying hypoxia often result in part from reduced chest wall movement due to pain, rather than from the pneumothorax.

10. F ★★★   OH Clin Surg, 4th edn → pp480–1

Oesophageal rupture should be considered in a patient developing haemothorax or pneumothorax after blunt chest trauma, in the absence of rib fractures. Mediastinal air is also frequently seen, and the presence of particulate matter in the chest drain is virtually pathognomonic.

→ http://www.facs.org/trauma/atls

11. G ★★★   OH Clin Surg, 4th edn → pp486–7

This patient's neurological findings are diagnostic of brain death, which under normal circumstances indicates no capacity for the recovery of central nervous system function. However, brain death should only be definitively diagnosed once hypothermia has been corrected ('you're not dead till you're warm and dead'); similarly, any pharmacological depression of consciousness must be redressed before confirming the diagnosis.

12. H ★★★★   OH Clin Surg, 4th edn → pp486–7

Skull fractures may be conservatively managed if the degree of depression is less than the thickness of the adjacent skull vault; overlying lacerations should be carefully washed and closed, and antibiotic prophylaxis prescribed. Significant skull fracture depression requires neurosurgical intervention.

13. B ★★   OH Clin Surg, 4th edn → pp486–7

The indications for CT scanning following head injury include reduced GCS 2h following the injury, loss of consciousness of more than 5min duration, significant retrograde amnesia, and suspected fracture to either the base or vault of the skull. This patient therefore does not immediately require CT; however, all patients showing signs of alcohol intoxication should be admitted for overnight head injury observations. The threshold for discharge should also be higher in the absence of a cohabitant who can closely observe the patient for signs of deterioration.

14. F ★★★   OH Clin Surg, 4th edn → pp486–7

Even in experienced hands, burr-hole craniostomy has an unacceptably high incidence of incorrect drill-hole placement, and should be avoided. Elevation of a bone flap is the treatment of choice for patients with intracranial mass lesions; this should be undertaken in the operating theatre environment by appropriately trained specialists.

15. C ★★   OH Clin Surg, 4th edn → pp486–7

Patients with no evidence of skull fracture whose GCS normalizes within 2h, who have no retrograde amnesia or focal neurology, and less than three episodes of vomiting may be discharged home provided another person will be at home to monitor for signs of neurological deterioration. All emergency departments should have printed advice for head injury patients and it should be ensured that the patient has understood this prior to discharge.

→ http://www.facs.org/trauma/atls

16. D ★ OH Clin Surg, 4th edn → pp478–9

Although this patient may well require both laparotomy and thoracotomy fairly urgently, establishment of an adequate airway remains the first priority, as with all trauma patients ('ABCDE').

17. H ★★★ OH Clin Surg, 4th edn → pp482–3

The absence of an exit wound is suggestive of deep penetrating bullet trauma to the abdomen. Even in the absence of high-grade shock, urgent exploratory laparotomy is indicated as the risk of visceral injury is high (approximately 90%).

18. H ★★★ OH Clin Surg, 4th edn → pp482–3

Air under the diaphragm following blunt abdominal trauma virtually confirms the presence of significant visceral injury and requires immediate laparotomy; the abdomen is also almost certainly the source of this patient's hypovolaemic shock. Other indications for emergency laparotomy following trauma include positive diagnostic peritoneal lavage, peritonitis, evisceration, and GI bleeding following sharp abdominal trauma.

19. A ★★★ OH Clin Surg, 4th edn → pp482–3

Trauma to solid intra-abdominal organs can be initially managed with close observation, provided the patient is haemodynamically stable and there is no evidence of intestinal or significant vascular injury. Frequent serial examinations are required to exclude development of signs of peritonism or shock, either of which would mandate urgent laparotomy.

20. G ★★★ OH Clin Surg, 4th edn → pp482–3

The presence of red cells is likely to be indicative of renal injury, although the paravertebral musculature often prevents significant damage to peritoneal or retroperitoneal structures from posterior stab wounds. If haemodynamically stable, such patients may be closely monitored without the automatic need for surgery; however, such monitoring should be undertaken in a hospital where on-site emergency surgical services are available, to allow any deterioration to be rapidly managed without the need for transfer.

→ http://www.facs.org/trauma/atls

Chapter 13

Orthopaedic surgery

Sebastian Dawson-Bowling

Sound knowledge of anatomy and understanding of musculoskeletal function underpins good orthopaedic practice. Bones and joints may be affected by genetic and degenerative conditions, by infection, primary and secondary neoplasia, by endocrine and metabolic anomalies, and by trauma.

As in other areas of surgery, a comprehensive history and thorough examination are essential in leading the clinician to a correct diagnosis. Appropriate imaging complements clinical acuity. The plain X-ray remains the primary modality of investigation for visualizing bony injuries and pathology, but MRI is a valuable adjunct for investigating soft tissues and joints.

Principles of fracture healing, reduction and fixation, and knowledge of consequences of complications which delay healing, or cause non-union, are integral to the practice of orthopaedic surgery.

This chapter will help you to revise basic tenets of orthopaedic practice and the common injuries and conditions encountered by the orthopaedic surgeon.

Frank Smith

QUESTIONS

Single Best Answers

1. A 77-year-old man falls down a flight of stairs sustaining injuries to the neck and right shoulder. In the emergency department he has tingling and weakness in his right arm. He is able to flex his elbow against gravity but cannot move it against resistance. Which *single* option is his Medical Research Council power grading? ★

A 0

B 1

C 2

D 3

E 4

2. An 80-year-old man falls onto his left side at home. His only past medical history is a previous inguinal hernia repair. On arrival in hospital his left leg is shortened and externally rotated. His pelvic radiograph is shown in Figure 13.1.

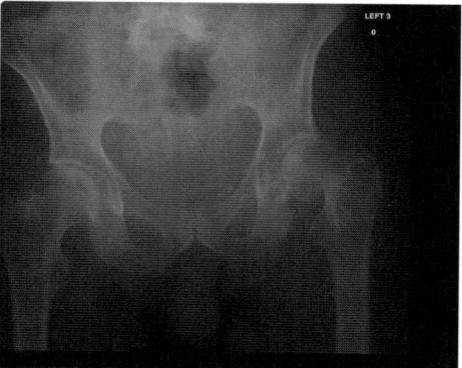

Figure 13.1 Pelvic radiograph

Which is the *single* most appropriate management of his injury? ★★

A Application of skin traction to left lower limb

B Left cannulated hip screw

C Left dynamic hip screw

D Left hip cephalomedullary nail

E Left hip hemiarthroplasty

3. An 82-year-old nursing home resident with severe ischaemic heart disease and dementia falls onto his non-dominant right hand and sustains the injury shown in Figure 13.2. The skin is intact and there is no distal neurovascular deficit.

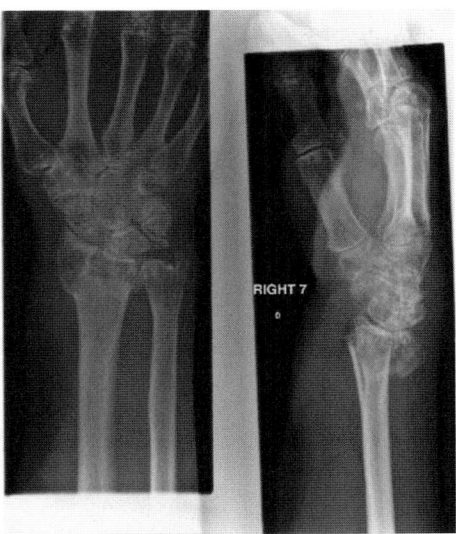

RIGHT 7

Figure 13.2 Injury to non-dominant right hand

Which is the *single* most appropriate initial treatment? ★★★

A Manipulation and cast immobilization

B Manipulation and K-wire fixation

C Open plate fixation via dorsal approach

D Open plate fixation via volar approach

E Primary wrist fusion

4. A 40-year-old woman attends the orthopaedic clinic with pain in her hands and legs. She also mentions that she has recently been feeling tired and depressed. Radiographs of her hands reveal cortical striations and subperiosteal bone resorption. Which is the *single* most likely diagnosis? ★

A Cervical spondylosis

B Hyperthyroidism

C Hyperparathyroidism

D Osteomalacia

E Osteoporosis

5. A 38-year-old farm labourer attends the emergency department, feeling generally unwell with pain in his shin. Eighteen months ago he sustained a grade II open fracture of his right lower leg, which was managed non-operatively. His temperature is 37.3°C, heart rate is 107bpm, and his right lower leg is swollen and erythematous. His investigations show: CRP 122mg/L and erythrocyte sedimentation rate 107mm/h. His radiograph is shown in Figure 13.3.

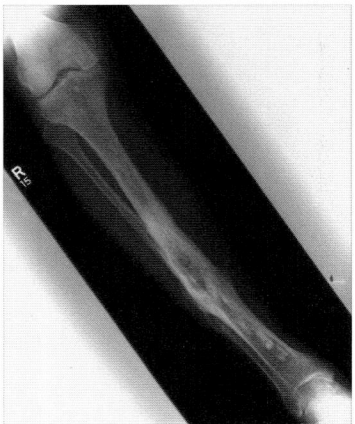

Figure 13.3 Radiograph of the patient

Which is the *single* most appropriate management? ★

A Below-knee amputation

B Intramedullary nailing

C IV flucloxacillin and observation

D Oral flucloxacillin with clinic follow-up at 2 weeks

E Surgical debridement

6. A 22-year-old barman trips and falls whilst carrying a drinks tray, sustaining a deep laceration to his right forearm from a shard of broken glass. Distal capillary refill time is 1sec, but he is found to have clawing and numbness of his ring and little fingers. When asked to grip a piece of paper in his first webspace, he does so by flexing his thumb interphalangeal joint. Which is the *single* most likely diagnosis? ★★★

A Median nerve neurotmesis

B Radial nerve axonotmesis

C Radial nerve neurapraxia

D Ulnar nerve axonotmesis

E Ulnar nerve neurotmesis

7. A 42-year-old woman falls down four stairs at home sustaining a closed injury to her left lower leg (radiograph shown in Figure 13.4). Her leg is put in a full fibreglass cast and she is admitted to the ward, pending operative fixation on the next trauma list. Four hours later she is screaming that she needs stronger painkillers.

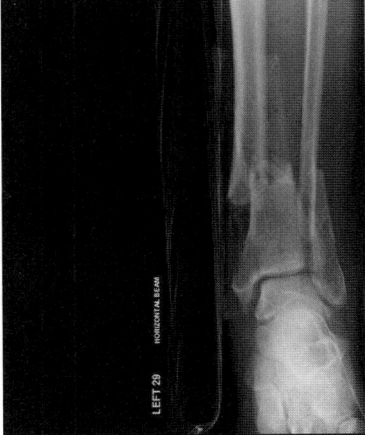

Figure 13.4 Radiograph of the left lower leg

Which is the *single* most appropriate next step in her management? ★

A Elevate limb above heart level and prescribe opioid analgesia

B Refer to anaesthetist for consideration of nerve block for overnight pain control

C Remove cast, elevate leg on a frame then clinically reassess

D Transfer immediately to theatre for emergency fasciotomy

E Transfer immediately to theatre for intramedullary nail fixation of fracture

8. A 47-year-old manual labourer attends the emergency department with worsening pain in his lumbar spine for 6 weeks. Which *single* clinical feature would suggest a diagnosis of discogenic pain? ★★★

A Pain is worse on bending forwards

B Pain is worse on lying flat

C Pain radiates to feet

D Presence of Waddell's signs

E Reduced Achilles tendon reflex

9. A 27-year-old man falls from a pushbike sustaining a wrist injury. His initial X-ray shows an isolated ulnar styloid fracture and the wrist is immobilized in plaster for 6 weeks. Two months later he returns to clinic with pain in the ulnar aspect of the wrist, worse on twisting and ulnar deviation. Repeat X-rays show the fracture to have united. Which is the *single* most likely diagnosis? ★★★★

A Perilunate dislocation

B Previously undiagnosed radial styloid fracture

C Previously undiagnosed scaphoid fracture

D Triangular fibrocartilage complex injury

E Ulnar neurapraxia

10. A 32-year-old orthopaedic registrar sustains a hand injury during the annual consultants versus juniors cricket match. His initial X-ray is shown in Figure 13.5.

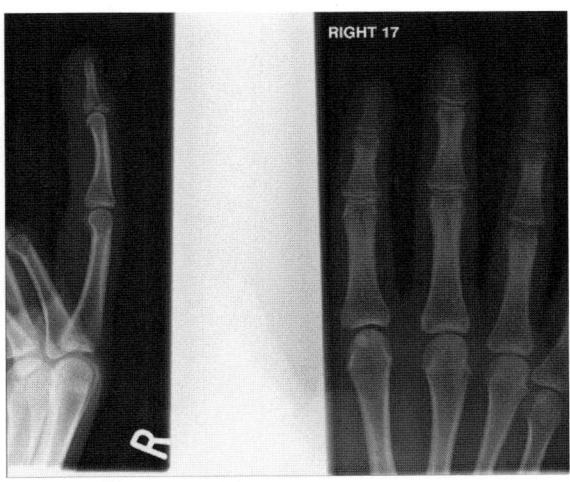

RIGHT 17

Figure 13.5 Initial X-ray of the patient

Which is the *single* most appropriate description of the injury seen? ★★

A Bennett's fracture

B Boxer's fracture

C Mallet injury

D Rolando fracture

E Schatzker injury

11. A 20-year-old gymnast falls onto her outstretched hand during a training session. In the emergency department she has pain in the elbow. Her X-ray is shown in Figure 13.6.

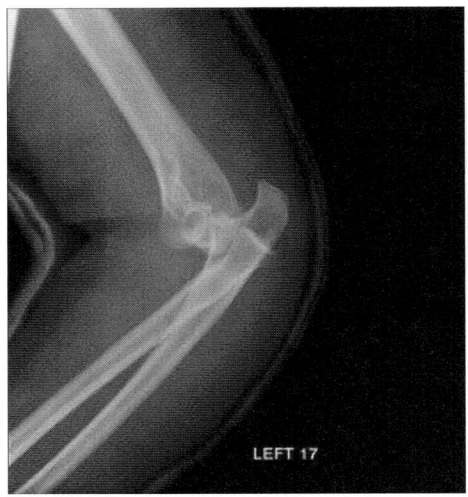

Figure 13.6 The X-ray of the patient's elbow

Which is the *single* most appropriate management? ★★★

A Plaster immobilization for 6 weeks followed by intensive physiotherapy

B Collar and cuff sling to allow gravity to effect a reduction

C K-wire fixation

D Open reduction and internal fixation

E Reduce under general anaesthetic

12. A 19-year-old woman falls from her horse sustaining an isolated injury to her right ankle. On arrival in hospital the ankle is swollen and obviously deformed; the hindfoot is tilted into a varus position and the lateral malleolus is clearly visible with some tenting of the overlying skin. Which is the *single* most appropriate next step in her management? ★★

A Immediate reduction and immobilization in the emergency department

B Immediate transfer to theatre for closed reduction under general anaesthesia

C Immediate transfer to theatre for open reduction under general anaesthesia

D Urgent Doppler ultrasound to assess dorsalis pedis pulse

E Urgent X-ray to assess bony injuries

13. A 23-year-old medical student crashes his motorbike into a roundabout at 50 miles per hour. He is brought to the emergency department by a passer-by, where the triage nurse arranges a single X-ray of his knee, shown in Figure 13.7.

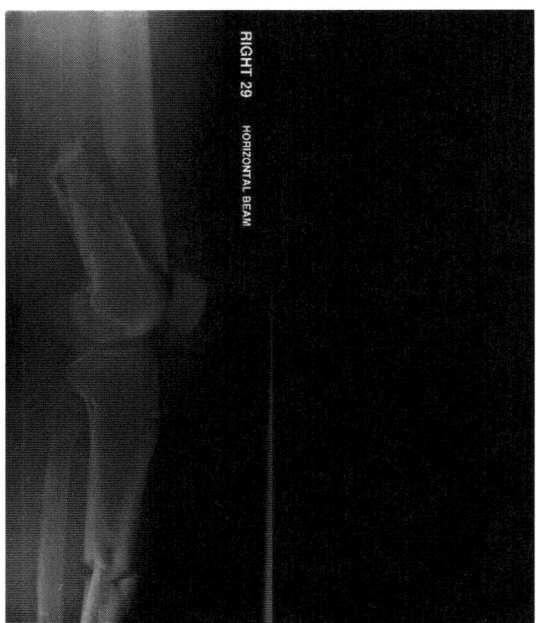

Figure 13.7 Single X-ray of the patient's knee

Which is the *single* most appropriate next step in his management? ★★

A Apply above-knee backslab before obtaining further imaging of whole lower limb to assess for further injuries

B Immobilize cervical spine and undertake formal primary survey according to ATLS protocol

C Obtain second radiograph at 90° to the first (i.e. anteroposterior view)

D Transfer urgently to theatre for retrograde intramedullary nail fixation of femur

E Undertake formal clinical examination of neck and limbs to exclude other skeletal injury

14. A 34-year-old partygoer falls off a balcony but is saved when his friends catch him by his right arm. A week later he attends the emergency department where his right upper limb is noted to be held in an internally rotated position, with the elbow extended, the forearm pronated and the wrist and fingers flexed. Which is the *single* most likely diagnosis? ★★

A Avulsion of long thoracic nerve of Bell

B Avulsion of suprascapular nerve

C Combined upper and lower brachial plexus injury

D Lower brachial plexus injury (Klumpke's palsy)

E Upper brachial plexus injury (Erb–Duchenne palsy)

15. A 42-year-old man loses control of his car and hits a tree at 40 miles per hour. He has bruising across his right shoulder and chest. He is assessed and managed according to ATLS protocol. No signs of cardiorespiratory or haemodynamic compromise are identified. His chest radiograph shows no evidence of pneumothorax or mediastinal injury; however, he is noted to have fractures of two ribs on the right side, and an undisplaced sternal fracture. No other injuries are identified. Which is the *single* most appropriate next step in his management? ★★★

A Admit for overnight cardiac monitoring

B Admit for planned rib fracture fixation on next available trauma list

C Discharge home for GP follow-up at 48h

D Insert chest drain for 48h

E Transfer urgently to theatre for fixation of his sternal fracture

16. A 32-year-old woman is admitted for elective right total hip replacement surgery. She has a history of untreated unilateral developmental dysplasia of the hip, as a result of which she has a pre-operative leg length discrepancy of 4cm. Her surgery is undertaken via an anterolateral approach without intraoperative complications, and the leg length is successfully restored. On the first operative day she is found to have a unilateral right-sided foot drop. Which is the *single* most likely cause for this clinical finding? ★★★★

A Division of sciatic nerve during initial surgical approach

B Intraoperative compression injury to common peroneal nerve due to over-inflation of tourniquet

C Long-standing neuropathy due to developmental dysplasia of the hip

D Postoperative development of thigh haematoma causing sciatic nerve compression in Hunter's canal

E Traction injury to sciatic nerve due to lengthening of limb

17. A 29-year-old man falls 15 feet from scaffolding whilst working on a building site. In the emergency department he is managed according to standard ATLS protocol. His abdomen is soft and non-tender, but there is blood at the urethral meatus and radiographs show displaced fractures of the right superior and inferior pubic rami, with a contralateral sacroiliac joint injury. No other injuries are identified. Following administration of 2L of crystalloid and 2 units of blood he remains haemodynamically unstable. Which is the *single* most appropriate next step in his management? ★★★

A Administer further transfusion of 4L of colloid further to assess haemodynamic status

B Apply circumferential compression with a sheet

C Arrange immediate transfer to a unit with facilities for undertaking pelvic trauma surgery

D Book urgent pelvic CT to clarify extent of injury to pelvic ring injury and allow planning of definitive surgery

E Transfer immediately to theatre for emergency laparotomy

18. A 71-year-old retired shopkeeper is referred with mild discomfort in her left wrist for 4 months, accompanied by development of a 0.5 × 0.5cm cystic swelling over the dorsal aspect of the joint. The swelling transilluminates, does not involve the overlying skin, has a rubbery consistency, and is minimally tender to touch. She has a full range of movement throughout the wrist and hand, and there is no distal neurovascular deficit. Radiographs show mild degenerative change throughout the wrist and carpus. Which is the *single* most appropriate next step in her management? ★★

A Add to elective waiting list for surgical excision

B Arrange urgent MRI to exclude synovial sarcoma

C Aspirate lesion in outpatient department using aseptic technique

D Inject the lesion with steroids in the outpatient department using aseptic technique

E Reassure and arrange follow-up appointment at 6 months

19. A 29-year-old man falls down a staircase at a nightclub, sustaining an isolated injury to his right ankle. On assessment in the emergency department the ankle is found to be deformed and swollen, with some tenting and discolouration of the overlying skin anteromedially. Perfusion of the toes is poor. His initial radiograph is shown in Figure 13.8.

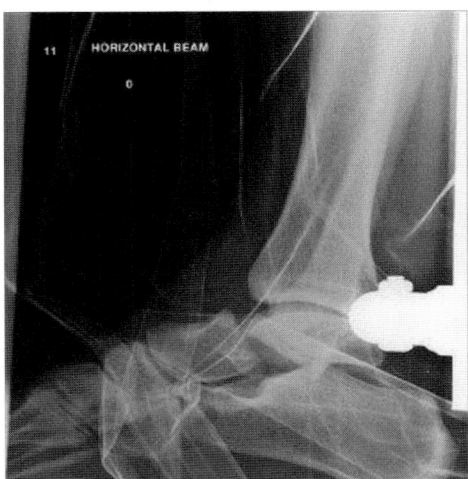

Figure 13.8 Initial radiograph of the patient's ankle

Which is the *single* most appropriate next step in his management?
★★★★

A Admit for overnight elevation and arrange open reduction and internal fixation of talus with screws on next morning's trauma list

B Admit for overnight elevation and arrange open reduction and internal fixation of os calcis with screws on next morning's trauma list

C Admit for overnight elevation then discharge in backslab with instructions to remain strictly non-weightbearing for 6 weeks

D Transfer to theatre as soon as possible for open reduction and internal fixation of talus with screws

E Transfer to theatre as soon as possible for open reduction and internal fixation of os calcis with screws

20. A 32-year-old man has had pain in his right thigh for 3 days, accompanied by feeling increasingly systemically unwell. He has sickle cell anaemia but is normally otherwise fit and well. On arrival in the emergency department his temperature is 38.1°C and his CRP is 92mg/L. An urgent ^{99}technetium bone scan suggests a diagnosis of acute osteomyelitis of the femur. Which is the *single* most likely causative organism? ★★

A *Enterococcus faecalis*

B *Escherichia coli*

C *Haemophilus influenzae* type b

D *Neisseria sp.*

E *Salmonella sp.*

ANSWERS

Single Best Answers

1. D ★   OH Clin Surg, 4th edn → p492

The Medical Research Council grading allows accurate documentation of motor function using a universal scoring system, although its critics point out that some of the grades represent a far wider spectrum of power levels than others. It is important to assess all muscle groups within the affected limb or myotomal distribution. The grading is shown in Table 13.1.

Table 13.1 Medical Research Council grading of motor function

Grade 0	No movement
Grade 1	Flicker of movement only
Grade 2	Movement with gravity eliminated
Grade 3	Movement against gravity
Grade 4	Movement against resistance
Grade 5	Normal power

2. E ★★   OH Clin Surg, 4th edn → p536

This patient has sustained a displaced intracapsular neck of femur fracture. Fixation with cannulated screws or dynamic hip screw is an option, but there is a high risk of subsequent failure and avascular necrosis of the femoral head. In a fit, active, fully compliant patient a total hip replacement is the best option. Despite a slightly increased risk of dislocation compared with hemiarthroplasty, outcome is improved. However, this is not an option here. An intramedullary nail which captures the femoral head is not generally used for intracapsular fractures. A hemiarthroplasty is the best choice to relieve pain and enable the patient to mobilize. Conservative management with skin traction carries high rates of morbidity due to prolonged immobilization.

3. A ★★★   OH Clin Surg, 4th edn → p510

These posteroanterior and lateral radiographs show a distal radius fracture. There is dorsal angulation and slight dorsal translation. It is not significantly shortened. There is an ulnar styloid fracture, but it is difficult to tell for sure if there is an intra-articular component to the fracture. However, if there is, the joint surface is congruent with no significant step. It is important to manage the patient and not the X-ray. In a young, fit patient one may well consider operative intervention for this injury. However, surgery in this patient would be risky and of questionable benefit to his functional outcome. An attempt at manipulation and a plaster cast is the best initial plan. If the position remains unacceptable or worsens, however, an operation may be necessary. Dorsal plating is associated with a high incidence of extensor tendon rupture and is rarely undertaken, and there is no role for primary wrist fusion in the management of distal radius fractures.

4. C ★   OH Clin Surg, 4th edn → p260

The classical presenting features of hyperparathyroidism may be remembered by the rhyme 'bones, stones, moans, and abdominal groans'. The characteristic radiological features are cortical striations and subperiosteal bone resorption in the phalanges. Cervical spondylosis refers to osteoarthritic change in the cervical spine. Osteomalacia (reduced bone mineralization) is characterized radiologically by the presence of Looser's zones (cortical defects) and blurring of the trabeculae. A diagnosis of osteoporosis cannot be made with a plain radiograph and bone densitometry scanning is required for definitive diagnosis. However, osteoporotic bone is often associated on plain X-ray with cortical thinning and reduced trabeculae. Hyperthyroidism does not cause specific changes to bone appearance, although osteoporosis is often present.

5. E ★   OH Clin Surg, 4th edn → p560

Chronic osteomyelitis may be seen as a sequela of trauma, especially to the lower leg, although the risk is reduced if the initial injury is treated with antibiotics and adequate debridement during the acute stage. This patient has features of systemic sepsis and the radiograph shows well-established osteomyelitic change; definitive surgical management is therefore required. Discharge home would be completely inappropriate. All sequestrum (infected dead bone) should be removed; serial debridement procedures may be required, potentially with subsequent plastic surgical intervention to achieve definitive soft tissue coverage. Antibiotic therapy is certainly indicated but is not the definitive management for this patient. Fixation may be required at the time of debridement or at a later stage but debridement is the priority at this stage. Although amputation may be a last resort in irretrievable cases, limb preservation should always be attempted and would be inappropriate in this scenario.

6. E ★★★★   OH Clin Surg, 4th edn → p564

A knowledge of the peripheral sensory and motor nerve distribution of the upper limb is essential in assessing such injuries. Low ulnar nerve injuries are characterized by clawing of the ulnar two digits, as well as a positive Froment's sign brought about by loss of innervation to the interossei (flexor pollicis longus is innervated by the anterior interosseous branch of the median nerve and therefore remains functional). Neurapraxia refers to temporary loss of conduction in a nerve due to stretching or compression, with no Wallerian (axonal) degeneration. Prognosis is excellent. Axonotmesis is characterized by degeneration of axons and myelin sheaths but not the surrounding connective tissue.

There is Wallerian degeneration and prognosis depends on the magnitude of injury. Neurotmesis involves complete disruption of all layers of the nerve. Wallerian degeneration is present. If surgical repair is successful axonal functional recovery occurs at 1mm per day. Prognosis is variable and age is the most important factor influencing successful recovery.

7. C ★   OH Clin Surg, 4th edn → p484

Compartment syndrome is common following fractures of the tibial shaft and a high index of suspicion is vital. Closed injuries have a higher risk than open injuries. Pain out of proportion to the injury, and pain on passive stretch of the compartments (flex and extend the great toe gently) should alert you immediately to this diagnosis. A backslab is preferable for temporary stabilization as it is less rigid than a full cast. If there is the slightest suspicion of compartment syndrome the cast must be split to the skin or removed immediately. Elevation is essential as well, but removing the constricting influence of the splint is the priority. Frequent clinical reassessment is required, and if signs and symptoms of compartment syndrome persist, early senior review is essential and fasciotomy should be considered. Intramedullary nailing is a common means of definitively stabilizing such fractures but will not treat compartment syndrome. Nerve blockade should never be used as it may mask symptoms of compartment syndrome.

8. A ★★★   OH Clin Surg, 4th edn → p578

Lumbar back pain is common, and in most cases self-limiting. A careful history and examination can help clarify the aetiology of the symptoms without automatic recourse to expensive imaging modalities. Exacerbation of pain on forward flexion is characteristic of discogenic pain, as opposed to facet joint arthropathy where pain is worse on extension of the spine. Reduced reflexes and radiation to the feet both suggest irritation of lumbar nerve roots as they pass through the exit foramina. Waddell described clinical signs characteristic of psychogenic (non-organic) back pain, although this should always be a diagnosis of exclusion.

9. D ★★★★   OH Clin Surg, 4th edn → p510

The triangular fibrocartilage complex is formed of the articular disc (triangular fibrocartilage), the ulnar ligaments of the wrist and the sheath of the extensor carpi ulnaris tendon. It is characteristically injured during compression with marked ulnar deviation, often with simultaneous fracture of the ulnar styloid. The clinical features are classically ulnar-sided wrist pain worse on ulnar deviation with or without rotation.

Ulnar neurapraxia would have resolved by 3.5 months post injury, and in event would present with altered sensation in the ulnar one-and-a-half digits. A fracture of the radial styloid is characterized by pain and tenderness at that site, and the scaphoid is on the radial side of the wrist. Perilunate dislocation is a severe acute injury in which multiple ligamentous tears allow the entire carpus to dislocate, leaving only the lunate in place.

10. C ★★   OH Clin Surg, 4th edn → p564

The mallet finger is characteristically a catching injury, and comprises detachment of the extensor tendon insertion from the distal phalanx, either with or without an associated bony fragment. The finger should be managed with 6 weeks of continuous immobilization in extension at the distal interphalangeal joint. A mallet splint is ideal for this.

Bennett's and Rolando fractures are both types of fracture dislocation of the base of the thumb; the Rolando having a more comminuted Y-type configuration. Schatzker classified fractures of the tibial plateau, but did not describe an eponymous hand injury. A boxer's fracture refers to a fracture of the 4th or more commonly 5th metacarpal neck, often sustained whilst punching a hard object.

11. E ★★★   OH Clin Surg, 4th edn → p522

Posterolateral elbow dislocation is reasonably common in young adults. Associated fractures are relatively infrequent, but thorough clinical and radiological assessment, particularly of the radial head and coronoid process, are mandatory; in children in particular, epicondylar or lateral condylar fracture must also be ruled out. In addition, injury to the brachial artery, ulnar nerve, and median nerve should be actively excluded.

Depending on local hospital policy regarding sedation, reduction can often be performed under sedation in the emergency department. If this is not possible reduction should be performed under general anaesthesia. Formal assessment of elbow stability is undertaken at the same time; medial collateral ligament injury, if present, is often associated with radial and coronoid fractures (the 'terrible triad').

Prolonged immobilization of a dislocated elbow is completely inappropriate. Immobilization of the elbow rapidly leads to stiffness and mobilization should start as early as possible. A dislocated elbow will not reduce spontaneously in a sling—this would be inappropriate management. In a simple dislocation such as this, there is no role for any form of operative fixation, either open or with K-wires.

12. A ★★   OH Clin Surg, 4th edn → p544

Displaced fracture dislocation of the ankle is an orthopaedic emergency, and is diagnosed clinically. The ankle should be immediately reduced before any imaging is obtained, to avoid the rapid development of skin necrosis that may otherwise develop, as well as possible neurovascular compromise or compartment syndrome. Imaging and definitive surgical treatment can then be planned in a more controlled fashion. Foot perfusion can be adequately assessed by clinical examination and there should be no need for Doppler ultrasound.

13. B ★★   OH Clin Surg, 4th edn → p538

Femoral shaft fractures frequently occur as part of polytrauma, especially in young patients. In such cases, particularly where there is a history of high-energy trauma, the patient should be formally managed according to standard ATLS protocol, with application of C-spine immobilization and oxygen, followed by a formal primary survey. Practically, several problems may be dealt with simultaneously, but a sequential approach should form the basis of the management strategy.

→ http://www.facs.org/trauma/atls

14. E ★★   OH Clin Surg, 4th edn → p566

The classic 'waiter's tip' deformity is diagnostic of an upper plexus injury affecting C5 and C6 ± C7. Klumpke's is characterized by clawing of the hand, which results from paralysis of the intrinsic muscles. Combined upper and lower plexus injuries are usually associated with significant trauma; all motor function in the affected limb is lost. Injury to the long thoracic nerve results in 'winging' of the scapula due to paralysis of serratus anterior.

15. A ★★★   OH Clin Surg, 4th edn → p530

Sternal and rib fractures almost always result from direct injuries, frequently from a seatbelt, when a characteristic bruise pattern may be seen. Rib fractures do not require operative intervention, but the presence of a sternal fracture is suggestive of a high-energy chest compression injury; close observation is required due to the risk of subsequent development of myocardial bruising and subsequent arrhythmia, cardiac tamponade or pneumothorax. A chest drain is only required in the presence of established haemothorax or pneumothorax.

16. E ★★★★   OH Clin Surg, 4th edn → p564

Sciatic nerve dysfunction is a recognized complication following correction of leg shortening in patients with developmental dysplasia of the hip; in general, it is not advisable to correct shortening by more than 2.5–3cm. Although the nerve can be injured during the surgical approach, this is associated with the posterior rather than anterolateral approach. Injury to the common peroneal nerve is reported, but normally results from blunt trauma from metal side supports during patient positioning. A tourniquet is not used during hip replacement surgery. The sciatic nerve does not pass through the subsartorial (Hunter's) canal. There is no neuropathy known to be associated with developmental dysplasia of the hip.

17. B ★★★   OH Clin Surg, 4th edn → p532

Severe haemodynamic instability frequently complicates pelvic trauma, due to concomitant vascular injury, most commonly to the iliac vessels; blood at the urethral meatus suggests simultaneous urogenital injury. In such cases, application of a pelvic external fixator often helps to tamponade the bleeding vessels—although this should be undertaken with caution where there is also posterior disruption to the pelvic ring. However, compression applied by circumferential application of a bedsheet is a very effective interim emergency measure for controlling bleeding. The sheet is tied round the level of the greater trochanters of the femurs to permit access to the abdomen and pelvis for subsequent surgery.

Transfer to either the CT scanner or a different unit is absolutely contraindicated in the haemodynamically unstable patient. Further fluid challenge without simultaneously addressing the source of bleeding is not indicated. There is no clinical suggestion of abdominal injury, so laparotomy is not indicated as a first-line treatment.

18. E ★★ OH Clin Surg, 4th edn → p577

The history and clinical findings are absolutely typical of a ganglion—a degenerative mucinous cyst arising from a joint or tendon sheath. Ninety per cent arise from either the volar or dorsal aspect of the wrist; of these, 50% resolve spontaneously, so patients should be persuaded where possible to opt for conservative management initially. Aspiration also gives an approximately 50% cure rate. Needle aspiration has a high recurrence rate so should not be encouraged. Surgery should only be undertaken if conservative measures fail, or if the lesion is compressing nearby neurovascular or other structures. Although MRI may be used where there is concern over possible malignancy, the clinical picture in this case does not suggest this.

19. D ★★★★ OH Clin Surg, 4th edn → pp498, 544

This may appear to be a difficult question requiring specialist orthopaedic knowledge, but it can be answered using basic principles. The skin is threatened, and the injury must therefore be reduced urgently. As such, any option to manage conservatively or wait till morning is incorrect. There is an artefact on the X-ray which appears to be a metallic object. However, a diagnosis is still possible. The radiograph clearly demonstrates a displaced fracture of the talar neck. This injury requires accurate open reduction and internal fixation due to the high risk of avascular necrosis (up to 90% even with operative treatment). The timing of surgery depends on the clinical picture—if there is significant swelling or evidence of compromise to the overlying skin, surgery should not be delayed until the next day. This patient's radiograph shows no evidence of a calcaneal injury, although further imaging would be required definitively to exclude this.

20. E ★★ OH Clin Surg, 4th edn → p558

Acute haematogenous osteomyelitis tends to occur in the epiphysis or metaphysis of growing bones (more commonly in boys than girls). There may be a history of a recent precipitating event such as a respiratory tract infection or cut to a nearby digit, but often this is not reported. Treatment should ideally be based on definitive identification of the causative organism, but where this is not possible, or will cause undue delay, a knowledge of the likely pathogen can help to guide empirical antimicrobial treatment.

Presentation in adulthood is rare without some form of immuno-compromise; in sickle patients the commonest organism is *Salmonella*; treatment should be with a fluoroquinolone or third-generation cephalosporin. *Escherichia coli* and *Haemophilus influenzae* type b are recognized causative organisms in infants and children respectively. *Neisseria* is found in sexually active adults.

Chapter 14

Plastic surgery

Olivier Branford

Principles of plastic surgery are integral to all surgical specialties. An understanding of wound healing, suture selection, skin closure, skin cover, and scar management forms an essential component of all modern surgical practice.

Appropriate assessment of burns and competent early management of the burned patient are prerequisite skills for all surgeons who work in emergency departments. However, transfer to and management in a specialist burns unit will ultimately result in the best outcome for these unfortunate patients. This forms one aspect of specialist plastic surgical practice.

The management of these and other conditions including soft tissue hand injuries, infections, and extensive skin loss through necrosis, whilst often requiring the skills of the specialist plastic surgeon, still form part of the broad general surgical curriculum.

This chapter will explore your understanding of the basic principles of plastic surgery which underpin the vast breadth of more specialist practice. The latter encompasses the complex multidisciplinary arenas of correction of birth defects and deformities, management of extensive traumatic injuries, cosmetic, and oncoplastic surgery.

Frank Smith

QUESTIONS

Single Best Answers

1. A 22-year-old man has a laceration to his left cheek following a fall. He has no other injuries. Which is the *single* most appropriate treatment in this case? ★★

A 2/0 or 3/0 suture, suture removal at 5–7 days

B 2/0 or 3/0 suture, suture removal at 14 days

C 3/0 or 4/0 suture, suture removal at 14 days

D 5/0 or 6/0 suture, suture removal at 5–7 days

E 5/0 or 6/0 suture, suture removal at 14 days

2. An 18-year-old woman has a defect on her upper back after removal of a dysplastic naevus. She is very keen to avoid an unsightly scar. Which is the *single* most appropriate treatment in this case? ★★

A Continuous suture

B Horizontal mattress suture

C Interrupted suture

D Subcuticular suture

E Vertical mattress suture

3. A 76-year-old woman is diagnosed with a pretibial haematoma, which is treated with evacuation and split skin grafting. The patient is otherwise fit and well and takes no regular medication. Her leg is cellulitic at the time of surgery. The graft is immobilized with quilting, foam dressing, and application of plaster of Paris to the affected limb. When checked at 5 days postoperatively the skin graft has not taken. Which is the *single* most likely cause? ★

A Haematoma

B Infection

C Non-suitable bed

D Seroma

E Shearing

4. A 57-year-old man has a full thickness skin graft to his forehead to reconstruct the defect following excision of a basal cell carcinoma. When checked at 5 days postoperatively the graft is adherent and appears viable. Which is the *single* most predominant stage of graft healing at this stage? ★★

A Fibrin adherence

B Lymphatic development

C Remodelling

D Revascularization

E Serum imbibition

5. A 38-year-old woman has a pedicled latissimus dorsi flap to reconstruct her breast following mastectomy. The patient is pain free and in a warmed room. Six hours postoperatively the flap is pale, cold, appearing 'underfilled', and has a prolonged capillary refill time with no bleeding on pin prick. Her pulse rate is 70bpm, her blood pressure is 125/65mmHg, and her urine output is 80mL/h. Which is the *single* most likely diagnosis? ★

A Arterial problem

B Nerve injury

C Haemorrhage

D Hypovolaemia

E Venous congestion

6. A 38-year-old woman has a firm, red, itchy raised scar following removal of a skin lesion from her sternum 3 months previously. The scar is confined to the boundaries of the original incision. She has tried scar massage and silicone gel but this is not helping. Which is the *single* most appropriate next line of treatment in this case? ★★

A Excision and closure

B Intralesional steroid injection

C Pulsed dye laser

D Radiotherapy

E Z-plasty

7. A 57-year-old man has an ulcerated, raised 7mm lesion on his right ear. It has bled spontaneously. Which is the *single* most likely diagnosis? ★★★

A Basal cell carcinoma

B Malignant eccrine poroma

C Malignant melanoma

D Microcystic adnexal carcinoma

E Squamous cell carcinoma

8. A 6-year-old girl has sustained a 16% hot water scald to her chest and arms after pulling a freshly boiled kettle onto herself. The burns are pink, blistered, and painful. Which is the *single* most accurate method for estimating the area of burn in this patient? ★★

A Assessing area of erythema

B Determining area of insensate skin

C Following a Lund and Browder chart

D Using examiner's hand as 1% of body surface

E Using the Wallace rule of nines

9. A 75-year-old man has suffered a 5% burn to his thighs from spilt hot tea. The burn is a blotchy red colour with bloody blisters, not blanching, and is sensate. There is fixed staining. Which is the *single* most likely type of burn this man has received? ★★

A Deep dermal burn

B Epidermal burn

C Full thickness burn

D Mid-dermal burn

E Superficial dermal burn

10. A 56-year-old man has sustained 8% deep dermal burns to his chest from a hot water scald. He has type 2 diabetes mellitus and had suffered myocardial infarction 1 year previously. He is carefully assessed, the burn washed, clingfilm applied, and adequate analgesia given. Which is the *single* most appropriate next step? ★★★

A Admit overnight for observation

B Discharge patient

C Fluid resuscitation

D Prepare patient for theatre

E Refer to a burns unit

11. A 32-year-old man has sustained 15% deep dermal burns to his face, neck, and upper anterior chest from hot oil catching fire in his kitchen. He is able to speak but is hoarse and breathless. He has singed nasal hairs and is coughing carbonaceous sputum. Which is the *single* most appropriate immediate management? ★

A Escharotomy

B Fluid resuscitation

C Immediate intubation

D Refer to burns unit

E Tangential burn excision

12. A 35-year-old woman has sustained a closed mallet injury to her left ring finger. A fracture fragment involving 20% of the distal interphalangeal joint articular surface is seen on the lateral radiograph. Which is the *single* most appropriate treatment? ★★★

A Open repair of extensor tendon

B Fracture fixation using Kirschner wire

C Manipulation of the joint under anaesthesia

D Mallet finger splint for 6 weeks

E Weekly examination with stress testing

13. A 19-year-old student has sustained a cat bite to her dominant right index finger. She has a sausage-like flexed index finger, pain on extension of her involved finger, and tenderness in her palm. Which is the *single* most likely diagnosis? ★★★

A Felon

B Flexor sheath infection

C Palmar space infection

D Paronychia

E Septic arthritis

14. A 46-year-old man has a rapidly progressive flexion deformity of his dominant left ring finger with contracture of his proximal interphalangeal joint. He is unable to place his hand flat on a table. His father and brother also have the same condition. The skin overlying the 4th ray in the palm is contracted and involved with the disease. He is otherwise fit and well. Which is the *single* most appropriate treatment? ★★★★

A Dermofasciectomy

B Limited fasciectomy

C Percutaneous fasciotomy

D Segmental fasciectomy

E Splintage only

15. A 32-year-old woman has neck pain, indentation of her shoulder skin from her bra straps, and difficulty in finding clothes that fit due to her 36GG breasts. She is requesting breast reduction. Which is the *single* most important consideration in drawing skin markings prior to surgery? ★★★

A Determining extent of glandular resection to achieve a specific BMI

B Determining extent of glandular resection to achieve a specific cup size

C Preservation of nipple blood supply and choice of skin excision pattern

D Preservation of nipple position and position of inframammary folds

E Preservation of nipple sensation and ability to breastfeed

16. A 24-year-old woman with a BMI of 19 kg/m^2 requests breast augmentation. Which is the *single* most appropriate positioning of the implants? ★★★★

A Inframammary

B Subcutaneous

C Submammary

D Under pectoralis major

E Under pectoralis minor

17. A 45-year-old woman is about to undergo mastectomy and is requesting immediate breast reconstruction. She has a good amount of abdominal skin and fat. She is keen to have autologous tissue only reconstruction and wants minimal donor site morbidity. Which is the *single* most appropriate treatment? ★★★★

A Deep inferior epigastric artery perforator flap

B Latissimus dorsi myocutaneous flap

C Subpectoral tissue expander

D Superior gluteal artery perforator flap

E Transverse rectus abdominis myocutaneous flap

Extended Matching Questions

Surgical flaps

For each scenario choose the *single* most appropriate flap from the list of options. Each option may be used once, more than once, or not at all.

A Bi-lobed flap

B Cross-leg flap

C Free fibular flap

D Free latissimus dorsi flap

E Gastrocnemius flap

F Pectoralis major flap

G Pedicled latissimus dorsi flap

H Rhomboid flap

I Rotation flap

1. A 23-year-old motorcyclist has a Gustilo and Anderson grade IIIB midshaft tibial fracture with a 10 × 18cm soft tissue defect. The orthopaedic surgeons have fixed the fracture with an intramedullary nail. ★★★★

2. A 76-year-old man has a basal cell carcinoma removed from his left temple. The 2.5cm defect will not close directly. ★★★★

3. A 53-year-old woman has a 6 × 8cm soft tissue defect over her left mandible with loss of the underlying bone following resection of a tumour. ★★★

4. A 68-year-old woman has a 4 × 6cm wound over her right knee, where her knee replacement prosthesis is visible. ★★★

5. A 75-year-old man has a 4 × 4cm full thickness scalp defect following excision of a basal cell carcinoma. ★★★

Excision of cutaneous lesions

For each scenario choose the *single* most appropriate type of excision from the list of options. Each option may be used once, more than once, or not at all.

A Circular excision, 4mm margin, with local flap

B Circular excision, 6mm margin, split skin graft

C Excision and direct closure, 1–2mm margin

D Excision and direct closure, 2–5mm margin

E Excision and direct closure, 10mm margin

F Incision biopsy including border of lesion

G Shave excision at mid-dermal level

H Wedge excision and closure

6. A 75-year-old man has a 6mm pearly nodular lesion on the helix of his ear, which has been present for 6 months. It bleeds and crusts but never disappears. ★

7. An 84-year-old woman has a 5mm greasy, oval, pigmented, verrucous lesion on her abdomen, which has been present for 3 years. It has a 'stuck-on' appearance. She is complaining that it is easily traumatized. ★★

8. A 23-year-old woman has a 3mm, round light brown lesion on her upper back which has not changed but she would like to have it removed as it catches on her bra. ★

9. A 69-year-old woman has a 23mm lesion with raised rolled edges on her right lower leg, which has a central ulcer and has been present for 6 weeks. ★★★

10. A 29-year-old man has an 11mm irregular, asymmetrical lesion on his upper back, which has a poorly defined edge. The lesion has increased in size over the last month. ★★

Soft tissue injuries

For each scenario choose the *single* most appropriate diagnosis from the list of options. Each option may be used once, more than once, or not at all.

A Extensor digitorum communis injury

B Extensor pollicis longus injury

C Flexor digitorum profundus injury

D Flexor digitorum superficialis injury

E Flexor pollicis longus injury

F Mallet injury

G Median nerve injury

H Ulnar collateral ligament injury

I Ulnar nerve injury

11. A 46-year-old woman has a laceration over the dorsum of her left wrist following a glass laceration. She is unable to retropulse her thumb and extend its interphalangeal joint. ★★

12. A 34-year-old man has sustained an injury to his thumb while skiing. The metacarpophalangeal joint of his thumb deviates radially on stress testing. ★★

13. A 46-year-old woman has sustained a knife injury to her left wrist. She has clawing of her hand. She is unable to abduct her fingers. ★

14. A 23-year-old rugby player sustains a closed injury to his index finger whilst grabbing another player's arm or shirt and is unable to flex his distal interphalangeal joint. ★★

15. A 19-year-old man has a glass laceration to his right wrist. He has weak thumb abduction. ★

ANSWERS

Single Best Answers

1. D ★★   OH Clin Surg, 4th edn → p590

The finest suture that is strong enough to maintain wound closure should be used. In the face this should be a 5/0 or 6/0 suture. In general, sutures should be removed at 5–7 days in a low-tension wound above the clavicle, and 7–14 days below it.

2. D ★★   OH Clin Surg, 4th edn → pp590–2

In order to prevent symptomatic, hypertrophic, and unsightly scars it is important to ensure that the skin incision is placed along relaxed skin tension lines where possible. The use of dermal sutures combined with a subcuticular running suture avoids suture marks, which would be seen with all the other suture techniques listed. Careful tension-free edge-to-edge closure with avoidance of dead space helps to improve the quality of the scar. Excessive use of deep dermal sutures is avoided to minimize any inflammatory response. Linear taping helps to flatten the scar both while the sutures are in place and for up to 2 months postoperatively. The patient is advised to massage the scar and to seek attention if the scar becomes hypertrophic for consideration of further treatment.

3. B ★   OH Clin Surg, 4th edn → pp594–5

In general, the most common cause of failure of graft take is haematoma. However, this patient's leg was cellulitic at the time of skin grafting. If there are more than 105 organisms per gram of tissue the skin graft will not take. Group A beta haemolytic *Streptococcus* is implicated in graft failure associated with cellulitis. The bacterial count must be reduced with debridement and antibiotics. It is advisable to confirm clinical improvement and microbiological confirmation of clear swabs prior to skin grafting in the cellulitic leg. Note that the causes of graft failure can easily be remembered with the acronym SHIN (shear/seroma, haematoma, infection, non-suitable bed).

4. D ★★   OH Clin Surg, 4th edn → pp594–5

The stages of graft take are fibrin adherence (immediate), serum imbibition (days 2–4) and revascularization (after day 4). Revascularization occurs either through one or more of the following: anastomosis between donor and recipient vessels (inoculation); ingrowth of vessels along channels of donor vessels; new vessel ingrowth (neovascularization). This is followed by lymphatic development, re-innervation, and remodelling.

5. A ★ OH Clin Surg, 4th edn → pp596–7

This patient's flap has the classic signs of an arterial problem. The five cardinal signs of acute arterial obstruction are: pain, pallor, pulselessness, paraesthesia, perishing with cold. Such situations need to be recognized promptly as good survival rates can be expected in flaps that are salvaged urgently in theatre by the plastic surgery team. Delays in identification and intervention result in proportionately poorer outcomes.

6. B ★★ OH Clin Surg, 4th edn → pp598–9

Intralesional steroid injection flattens hypertrophic scars and may reduce scar symptoms such as pain and itching. Repeated injections are required at 6- to 8-week intervals. Cytotoxics, such as fluorouracil, may also be used. Silicone gel, tape, or sheets reduce hypertrophy and relieve itch and may be used in combination with other treatments. Laser can be useful in reducing pigmentation and inflammation. Radiotherapy is effective but should be reserved for patients known to be prone to hypertrophic or keloid scarring and is given as a course of five or six doses beginning within 24h following scar excision. Further surgery should be avoided for at least 6 months, until the scar is mature, unless it is causing a contracture. The scar is likely to recur if surgery is used alone.

7. E ★★★ OH Clin Surg, 4th edn → pp602–3

The most common skin cancer overall is basal cell carcinoma. The most common skin cancer involving the ear is squamous cell carcinoma. Although this is classically described as being a raised, rolled lesion with a central ulcer, it may also present as an indurated and nodular lesion, a scaly erythematous patch, or a non-raised non-healing ulcer. Basal cell carcinomas have a rolled pearly edge and small visible blood vessels. Some basal cell carcinomas are pigmented, flat, and scaly, with a waxy appearance and an indistinct border.

The intraepidermal portion of the eccrine gland can give rise to a benign eccrine poroma which although rare can turn malignant but should be suspected in patients who present with pain, bleeding, and itching.

Microcystic adnexal carcinoma is a tumour of the skin appendage which is typically a sweat gland carcinoma. They are common on the head, neck, and especially the face. It invades locally quite aggressively but hardly metastasizes.

8. C ★★ OH Clin Surg, 4th edn → pp604–5

The rule of nines does not apply to children as they have disproportionately large heads and small limbs relative to adults. Skin erythema and sensation are used to assess burn depth. Erythema is not included in the assessment when determining fluid requirement. It is the patient's hand, and not the examiner's that represents 1% total body surface area.

9. A ★★ OH Clin Surg, 4th edn → pp604–5

Burn degrees are described in Table 14.1.

Table 14.1 Degrees of burns

First degree (epidermal burn)	Erythema, dry, and painful
Second degree (superficial partial thickness—extends into superficial dermis)	Red with clear blisters, blanches with pressure, moist, painful
Second degree (deep partial thickness—extends into deep dermis)	Red and white with bloody blisters, less blanching, moist, and painful
Third degree (full thickness—extends through entire dermis)	Stiff and white/brown, dry, leathery, painless
Fourth degree (extends through skin, subcutaneous tissue, muscle, and bone)	Black, charred with eschar, painless

10. E ★★★   OH Clin Surg, 4th edn → pp606–7

According to guidance from the National Burn Care Review, this patient meets the criteria for referral to a burns unit due to his comorbidities. Burn patients are referred based on the complexity of their injury. Patients requiring referral include those aged under 5 years or over 60 years, those with flexural burns, circumferential limb and chest burns, or those burns involving the face, hands, perineum, or feet. Chemical burns and other specific mechanisms of injury should also be referred. Inhalational injury should always be referred after appropriate airway management. Paediatric burns greater than 5% total body surface area, or 10% in those aged 16 or over are also referred. Patients with certain comorbidities such as diabetes or myocardial infarction within the last 5 years should be referred to a burns unit, as should any burn associated with major trauma.

→ http://www.nbcg.nhs.uk/national-burn-care-review

11. C ★   OH Clin Surg, 4th edn → pp606–9

This patient has the signs of impending airway obstruction, requiring humidified 100% oxygen and immediate intubation. He may also have oropharyngeal burns and a blistered palate. He will require fluid resuscitation and transfer for further management in a burns unit once his airway is secure. Escharotomy is indicated in circumferential full thickness burns to the chest.

→ http://www.specialisedservices.nhs.uk/library/35/National_Burn_Care_Referral_Guidance.pdf

12. D ★★★   OH Clin Surg, 4th edn → pp504, 610

Most mallet injuries are treated with immobilization of the distal interphalangeal joint in extension. This extension should be maintained without even a momentary lapse for 6–8 weeks in continuous splinting. Tendinous injuries require 6–8 weeks of splinting, and bony injuries require 6 weeks. Mallet injuries that are accompanied by volar subluxation of the distal phalanx are usually treated surgically. The belief is that restoring joint alignment and the balance between flexor and extensor forces is needed to obtain an adequate functional result in these patients. The joint is reduced and a transarticular Kirschner wire (K-wire) is placed.

13. B ★★★   OH Clin Surg, 4th edn → p612

This patient has the classic signs of flexor sheath infection as first described by Kanavel. The four cardinal signs are: flexed posture of the involved finger, pain on passive extension, fusiform digital swelling, and pain along the flexor sheath in the palm. This is a plastic surgical emergency and must be treated with surgical exploration, drainage of pus, washout of the flexor sheath, and IV antibiotics if stiffness and contractures are to be avoided. Cat bites are likely to be infected with *Pasteurella multocida* and are best treated with intravenous co-amoxiclav unless the patient is allergic to penicillin.

Felon is an abscess of the terminal pulp space of the finger as a consequence of penetrating trauma which gives rise to secondary infection.

Paronychia is a common infection that commences from beneath the eponychium arising from a hang nail or manicurist's instrument. Suppuration ensues which then advances around the nail fold and burrows beneath the base of the nail (subungual abscess).

→ Draeger RW, Bynum DK Jr. Flexor tendon sheath infections of the hand. *J Am Acad Orthop Surg* 2012; 20(6):373–82.

14. A ★★★★   OH Clin Surg, 4th edn → pp614–15

This patient has Dupuytren's disease (Figure 14.1). The ring finger is usually the first to be affected. Aetiology is unknown but there is often a higher incidence amongst relatives. Surgery is indicated when there is metacarpophalangeal joint fixed flexion contracture of more than 30°, any proximal interphalangeal joint contracture, any rapidly progressing contractures, or when the hand will not lie flat on a table. This patient requires surgery, with excision of the involved skin to act as a 'firebreak' to reduce recurrence, and full thickness skin grafting of the resultant defect.

15. C ★★★   OH Clin Surg, 4th edn → p616

The general principle of breast reduction surgery is to reduce both the skin envelope and the substance of the breast to create a smaller, more pert breast with the nipple and the areola lying higher than they currently do.

The two main operative considerations are:

- Maintaining the blood supply to the nipple using a superomedial, superior, inferior, lateral or central pedicle.
- The nature of the skin excision pattern (inverted 'T'-shaped, peri-areolar incision only, peri-areolar incision with vertical scar) which determines the location of the final scars. This results in significant scar formation over the breast, which is absolutely impossible to avoid.

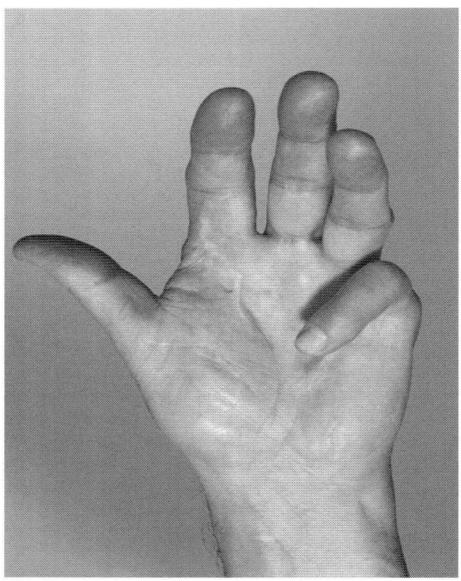

Figure 14.1 Dupuytren's disease
Reproduced from Longmore et al., *Oxford Handbook of Clinical Medicine*, 8th edition, 2010, with permission from Oxford University Press.

The aim is also simply to make the bust size more in proportion with the overall frame and figure of the patient. Many women notice altered sensation around the nipple and the areola and around the scars in the breast. The sensation is normally reduced to some extent but for some women it may actually be increased or even be oversensitive. The nipple is elevated during breast reduction. Most women will not be able to breastfeed after the operation.

16. D ★★★★ OH Clin Surg, 4th edn → p618

Breast implants are placed either in the submammary (under the breast tissue and above pectoralis major) or subpectoral (below pectoralis major) positions. Breast augmentation in submammary position in thin patients may cause rippling, palpability, and visibility of the implant due to the lack of breast tissue coverage. Thin patients are an indication for submuscular implant placement. This technique can offer a high-grade result especially in thin patients with less subcutaneous tissue, it provides excellent upper and lower pole coverage and gives the shape of the breast a natural appearance, with no palpability or rippling. There is no consensus on which position is better but it is generally accepted that subpectoral implant on a very thin patient as described in the scenario would have better results.

17. A ★★★★   OH Clin Surg, 4th edn → p618

Subpectoral tissue expanders either remain *in situ* or are replaced with implants, with the attendant risk of capsule formation and the need for further surgery. The transverse rectus abdominis myocutaneous flap procedure uses tissue and muscle from the lower abdominal wall. The skin, fat, blood vessels, and at least one abdominal muscle are harvested from the abdomen and moved to the chest. There is a 5% risk of abdominal hernias or bulges with a transverse rectus abdominis myocutaneous flap. Deep inferior epigastric artery perforator flap uses fat and skin from the same area as in the transverse rectus abdominis myocutaneous flap but does not use the muscle to form the breast mound. This results in less skin and fat in the lower abdomen, or a 'tummy tuck' and it reduces donor site morbidity with less muscle weakness and fewer hernias. Latissimus dorsi flap is made up of skin, fat, muscle, and blood vessels from the upper back. It is tunnelled under the skin to the front of the chest. Some women may have weakness in their back, shoulder, or arm after this surgery. Gluteal free (gluteal artery perforator) flap is a newer type of surgery that uses tissue from the buttocks, including the gluteal muscle, to create the breast shape. It is an option for women who cannot or do not wish to use the tummy sites due to thinness, incisions, failed tummy flap.

Extended Matching Questions

1. D ★★★★   OH Clin Surg, 4th edn → pp596–7

Gustilo-Anderson grade IIIB fracture is a highly contaminated, comminuted, greater than 10cm wound with severe soft tissue injury usually needing reconstructive surgery for coverage.

This large defect requires a large flap. As internal fixation has been performed it is important to achieve adequate soft tissue coverage at the same time as insertion of the implant in an orthoplastic approach. The latissimus dorsi flap is a reliable flap with a long pedicle which gives it the advantage of keeping the anastomosis out of the zone of injury. It is very useful in large traumatic wounds.

2. H ★★★★   OH Clin Surg, 4th edn → pp596–7

The rhomboid flap is well suited to temple defects, where skin laxity exists adjacent to the defect. The rhomboid flap orientation should be such that the donor scar is placed in the relaxed skin tension lines.

3. C ★★★ OH Clin Surg, 4th edn → pp596–7

The free fibular flap can be raised with skin, muscle, and bone and is a good choice for reconstructing the mandible. The flap has the advantage of having little donor site morbidity.

4. E ★★★ OH Clin Surg, 4th edn → pp596–7

The pedicled gastrocnemius flap is a good choice for defects around the knee. The medial head of gastrocnemius is usually chosen over the lateral head as it has greater muscle bulk and length. The flap is skin grafted after transfer.

5. I ★★★ OH Clin Surg, 4th edn → pp596–7

In this patient a scalp rotation flap may be used. This is a semi-circular flap which is rotated into the defect about the pivot point.

6. H ★ OH Clin Surg, 4th edn → pp602–3

The description of this lesion is typical of a basal cell carcinoma, which occurs most commonly in the head and neck region. The helix of the ear is best treated with a wedge excision, which maintains the shape of the ear, although this is reduced in size.

7. G ★★ OH Clin Surg, 4th edn → pp600–1

This description is typical of a seborrhoeic keratosis, which are more common with increasing age. These are best treated with shave excision, although the specimens should be sent for histology as 1 in 16 may be a malignant tumour. If the specimen shows malignancy then depending on the type of malignancy and the involvement of the margins re-excision may be indicated.

8. C ★ OH Clin Surg, 4th edn → pp600–1

This lesion is likely to be benign and only requires a minimal excision margin of 1–2 mm. The lines of relaxed skin tension should be used as the long axis of the excision.

9. B ★★★ OH Clin Surg, 4th edn → pp602–3

This lesion has the typical features of a squamous cell carcinoma. It is over 2cm in diameter and should therefore be excised with a 6mm margin as it is a high-risk lesion.

The lower leg in older female patients has thin skin with little laxity and is unlikely to be suitable for direct closure. The resultant defect is likely to require a split thickness skin graft.

→ http://www.bad.org.uk/Portals/_Bad/Guidelines/Clinical%20 Guidelines/SCC%20Guidelines%20Final%20Aug%2009.pdf

10. D ★★ OH Clin Surg, 4th edn → pp602–3

This lesion has the features of a malignant melanoma. The short history of an increase in size, combined with the irregular, poorly defined appearance make urgent excision mandatory, with a recommended 2–5mm margin, to obtain the diagnosis and assessment of Breslow thickness to guide further treatment.

11. B ★★ OH Clin Surg, 4th edn → pp504, 610

The extensor pollicis longus tendon extends the thumb dorsal to the plane of the hand, allowing a patient with the palm flat on a table to lift the thumb.

12. H ★★ OH Clin Surg, 4th edn → p564

An acute ulnar collateral ligament injury of the thumb is common among skiers (skier's thumb) and is suspected by pain and laxity when the thumb metacarpophalangeal joint is stressed radially.

13. I ★ OH Clin Surg, 4th edn → p610

This patient may also have numbness in the ulnar one-and-a-half digits. The ulnar nerve supplies all the intrinsic muscles of the hand except the lateral two lumbricals, opponens pollicis, abductor pollicis brevis, and flexor pollicis brevis (LOAF) muscles. Clawing is the result of unopposed action of the long extensors on the metacarpophalangeal joint and unopposed action of the long flexors on the interphalangeal joints. Paralysis of the interossei results in absent finger abduction.

14. C ★★ OH Clin Surg, 4th edn → p610

Jersey finger is a closed injury to the flexor digitorum profundus tendon at its insertion to the distal phalanx, resulting from hyperextension.

15. G ★ OH Clin Surg, 4th edn → pp505, 610

This patient may also have numbness in the radial three-and-a-half digits. The muscles of the hand supplied by the median nerve are the lateral two lumbricals, opponens pollicis, abductor pollicis brevis, and flexor pollicis brevis (LOAF).

Chapter 15

Cardiothoracic surgery

Olivier Branford and Simon Fisher

Management of the cardiothoracic patient is diagnostically and technically demanding. Cardiothoracic surgery comprises cardiac and thoracic components. Whilst overlap exists between treatment of pulmonary conditions including lung neoplasia, infection and ventilatory dysfunction, and treatment of cardiac disease, progressively surgeons tend to specialize in one area or the other.

Boundaries between cardiac surgery and interventional cardiology are also diminishing as new endovascular interventions—for instance, in coronary artery angioplasty, stenting, and valve replacement—achieve growing therapeutic prominence and compete with open surgical procedures.

A firm grasp of cardiopulmonary physiology underpins understanding of cardiovascular function and of the pathologies affecting these systems. This chapter will test you on aspects of pulmonary pathology, cardiovascular physiology, and on ischaemic heart disease and valvular dysfunction. This should help you to revise key aspects in this demanding and rapidly evolving area of surgery.

Frank Smith

QUESTIONS

Single Best Answers

1. A 62-year-old woman with a 45-pack-year history has lost 5kg, has developed a left-sided ptosis, a constricted pupil on the same side, and has a persistent cough. She has a pleural effusion. Which is the *single* most likely diagnosis? ★★

A Bronchial adenocarcinoma

B Bronchial squamous cell carcinoma

C Large cell undifferentiated carcinoma

D Meigs' syndrome

E Small cell carcinoma

2. A 56-year-old heating engineer recently returned from a holiday in Egypt has haematuria and haemoptysis. He is cachectic and has bilateral pleural effusions. Which is the *single* most likely diagnosis? ★★★

A Mesothelioma and renal cell carcinoma

B Prostate cancer and urinary tract obstruction

C Schistosomiasis and liver fibrosis

D Seminoma and lung metastases

E Tuberculosis

3. A 55-year-old woman with a 30-pack-year history has developed a right pleural effusion, confirmed by erect posteroanterior chest X-ray. No other abnormality is seen. Which is the *single* most appropriate management? ★★★★

A CT scan

B Thoracocentesis with aspirate sent for protein, albumin, amylase, pH, glucose, Gram stain and culture, white cell count, cytology

C Thoracocentesis with aspirate sent for Light's criteria, albumin, amylase, pH, glucose, Gram stain and culture, white cell count, cytology plus serum sent for protein, albumin, and glucose

D Thoracocentesis with aspirate sent for Light's criteria, albumin, amylase, pH, glucose, Gram stain and culture, white cell count, cytology plus serum sent for protein, LDH, albumin, and glucose

E Thoracocentesis with aspirate sent for protein, albumin, amylase, pH, glucose, Gram stain and culture, white cell count, cytology plus serum sent for protein, albumin, and glucose

4. A 19-year-old man has blunt chest trauma following a road traffic collision. His heart rate is 130bpm, blood pressure is 85/60mmHg, respiratory rate is 30/min. His airway is clear, his jugular venous pressure is raised, and heart sounds are muffled. Primary survey has found no other injuries. ECG shows multiple ectopic beats. Two large bore IV cannulae are placed and IV fluid administration commenced. Which is the *single* most appropriate next step? ★★

A Amiodarone infusion

B Insertion of chest drain

C Obtain cervical spinal X-rays

D Obtain chest X-ray

E Pericardiocentesis

5. A 24-year-old woman with cystic fibrosis has developed increased dyspnoea and sudden onset right pleuritic chest pain. Her heart rate is 98bpm, blood pressure is 160/85mmHg, respiratory rate is 25/min, and SaO_2 88% on air. Her trachea is central with no tug and apex beat is in the 5th intercostal space in the mid-clavicular line. Percussion of the right chest demonstrates hyperresonance. Which is the *single* most appropriate next step? ★

A Administer oxygen by facemask

B Needle thoracocentesis

C Obtain arterial blood gas

D Obtain chest X-ray

E Right-sided chest drain insertion

6. An 18-year-old man in the emergency department has sustained a traumatic pneumothorax and has had a chest drain inserted. After initially stabilizing, his heart rate has risen to 110bpm. Respiratory rate is 28/min and SaO_2 has fallen to 90% on oxygen administered at 12L/min. The anaesthetist is satisfied with the airway position. Which is the *single* most appropriate next step? ★

A Administer diuretics

B Repeat chest X-ray

C Repeat chest examination

D Repeat survey for haemorrhage

E Replace chest drain

7. A 75-year-old man who has had a previous myocardial infarction undergoes preoperative echocardiography to assess his cardiac function prior to open abdominal aortic aneurysm repair. The consultant anaesthetist in the pre-assessment clinic is asked to provide some revision teaching of cardiac physiology. Which *single* statement with respect to the patient's cardiovascular parameters is correct? ★

A Cardiac index represents stroke volume divided by cardiac output

B Left atrial pressure is an indirect measure of afterload

C Left ventricular end-diastolic pressure is an indirect measure of compliance

D Mean arterial pressure is half the difference between systolic and diastolic arterial pressure, added to diastolic pressure

E Systemic vascular resistance is an indirect measure of preload

8. A 68-year-old man has central chest pain radiating to his left arm during mild exertion on treadmill testing. He is referred for coronary angiography which demonstrates triple vessel disease with >70% stenosis and is listed for coronary artery bypass grafting (CABG). A medical student asks for teaching with respect to coronary bypass surgery. Which *single* statement is correct? ★★★

A Cardioplegia is used in CABG to stop the beating heart by cooling

B Cardiopulmonary bypass involves oxygenation of blood derived via an aortic cannula, returned by the circuit to the right atrium

C Long saphenous vein grafts to the left anterior descending coronary artery have superior long-term patency compared to other conduits

D On completion of CABG, the effects of therapeutic heparin are reversed by protamine

E The right internal mammary artery is one of the three most commonly used conduits for CABG

9. A 45-year-old woman with myasthenia gravis undergoes a thoracic CT scan which demonstrates a thymoma. Thymectomy via median sternotomy is planned. A medical student asks the thoracic surgeon to explain the relevant anatomy. Which *single* statement is correct? ★★

A The anterior mediastinum extends from the thoracic inlet to the line between the sternal angle and the T4–5 space

B The phrenic nerves are contained in the posterior mediastinum

C The thoracic duct is contained in the posterior and superior mediastinum

D The thymus is contained in the superior mediastinum

E The thymus is a lymphoid structure which takes over production of T cells in later life

Extended Matching Questions

EMQ 1

For each scenario choose the *single* most likely diagnosis from the list of options. Each option may be used once, more than once, or not at all.

A Bronchial adenocarcinoma

B Mesothelioma

C Pancoast's tumour

D Pneumonia

E Pneumothorax

F Pulmonary embolus

G Pulmonary oedema

H Ruptured left main bronchus

I Squamous cell bronchial carcinoma

1. A 56-year-old woman has haemoptysis, severe pleuritic chest pain, and shortness of breath. She takes hormone replacement therapy, has a 20-pack-year history, and has recently visited relatives in Australia. ★

2. An 84-year-old man has shortness of breath, orthopnoea, and paroxysmal nocturnal dyspnoea with bilateral pitting oedema of the ankles. He has developed a cough with frothy pink sputum. ★

3. A 67-year-old housewife has haemoptysis and dyspnoea. Her husband was employed for many years as a demolition worker and was exposed to asbestos. ★★

4. A 25-year-old man with a BMI of 16 and a 13-pack-year history has developed sharp inspiratory pain with reduced chest wall movement on the left and quiet breath sounds in the same region. ★

5. A 59-year-old shop manager with a 32-pack-year history has lost one and a half stones over the past 3 months and has blood-streaked purulent sputum with progressive stridor. ★

EMQ 2

For each scenario choose the *single* most likely diagnosis from the list of options. Each option may be used once, more than once, or not at all.

A Aortic regurgitation

B Aortic stenosis

C Hepatitis

D Mitral valve regurgitation

E Mitral valve stenosis

F Mitral valve vegetation

G Paravalvular leak

H Prosthetic mitral valve embolus

I Pulmonary valve vegetation

J Ruptured papillary muscle

K Tricuspid insufficiency

6. A 26-year-old IV drug user with a recurrent pneumonia has developed a mid-diastolic murmur. ★★

7. A 62-year-old man has jaundice, raised jugular venous pressure, a pansystolic murmur, and pulsatile varicose veins. ★★

8. A 57-year-old man who had rheumatic fever in childhood has a prosthetic mitral valve. He has recently become jaundiced, has a pansystolic murmur, and haemoglobin of 9.5g/dL. ★★

9. A 54-year-old man was recently admitted to the coronary care unit and underwent coronary thrombolysis following acute onset chest pain. He now has exertional dyspnoea, oedematous ankles, and a pansystolic murmur. ★★

10. A 78-year-old man with a history of transient ischaemic attacks and a recent collapse is seen in the vascular clinic for carotid artery assessment. He has shortness of breath, a slow rising pulse, and a systolic murmur with bilateral carotid bruits. ★★★

ANSWERS

Single Best Answers

1. E ★★   OH Clin Surg, 4th edn → p632

Small cell carcinoma—this neuroendocrine tumour comprises approximately 20% of bronchial tumours. Small cell carcinomas are the most common Pancoast's tumours, i.e. tumours found at the apex of the lung, which infiltrate the adjacent ribs compressing the sympathetic ganglion resulting in an ipsilateral Horner's syndrome. Meigs' syndrome comprises ascites and pleural effusions associated with benign ovarian tumours. Squamous cell carcinoma is the most common lung tumour in Europe, often arising as an endobronchial mass in large airways. Both adenocarcinoma and large cell undifferentiated carcinoma are more likely to occur as peripheral tumours and unlikely to compress the sympathetic ganglion.

2. A ★★★   OH Clin Surg, 4th edn → p632

Occupational exposure to asbestos is associated with both mesothelioma and renal cell carcinoma. Prostate cancer may cause lower urinary tract symptoms and haematuria, but spreads by direct invasion or metastatic spread to bone or to local lymph nodes, and not usually to the lungs. Schistosomiasis (bilharziasis) is a parasitic disease of the urinary and GI tracts prevalent in tropical regions of Africa and Asia, which may cause periportal liver fibrosis. Rarely, systemic infection of the lungs may cause dyspnoea but the temporal relationship of possible exposure to parasites and liver fibrosis makes this diagnosis unlikely in this case and would not explain haemoptysis. Seminomas are testicular tumours which may metastasize to para-aortic lymph nodes and by haematogenous spread to the lungs, but do not involve the urinary tract. Tuberculosis may affect both respiratory and renal tracts but is not suggested by the history of a recent holiday in this case and is not associated with asbestos exposure.

3. D ★★★★   OH Clin Surg, 4th edn → p634

Light's criteria, (Light et al., 1972), compare pleural fluid protein and LDH with that of serum, differentiating between patients with exudates and transudates. The other biochemical tests improve the accuracy of this definition with the exception of glucose. Glucose and the microbiology tests identify infection. Cytology tests are aimed at confirming malignancy. CT scan is not indicated prior to the investigations described.

→ Light R, MacGregor M, Luchsinger P, Ball W. Pleural effusions: the diagnostic separation of transudates and exudates. *Ann Intern Med* 1972; **77**(4):507–13.

4. E ★★   OH Clin Surg, 4th edn → p638

This patient is displaying Beck's triad (Claude Beck, pioneer American heart surgeon) of raised jugular venous pressure, muffled heart sounds, and low blood pressure. He has a mechanism of injury compatible with cardiac tamponade. He requires definitive intervention, pericardiocentesis, plus IV fluids to improve his venous return and improve his cardiac output. Amiodarone may be considered later. A chest X-ray may show his pericardial effusion but will delay critical intervention. There are no clinical signs of haemopneumothorax to suggest the need for urgent chest drainage prior to chest X-ray.

It should be noted that the role of needle pericardiocentesis is controversial. The procedure may be ineffective at removing clotted blood within the pericardium and is not without risk of injury to the coronary arteries. Where circumstances permit, in established cardiac tamponade, urgent formal surgical pericardotomy may be more appropriate.

5. A ★   OH Clin Surg, 4th edn → pp480, 638

This patient has not been adequately resuscitated yet, her pneumothorax and dyspnoea are compromising oxygenation on room air and so her inspired oxygen concentration must be increased. At this stage an arterial blood gas is not necessary. There is no clinical indication of tension pneumothorax and so decompression by needle thoracocentesis is not required. A chest X-ray would confirm a simple pneumothorax and then a chest drain could be inserted.

6. C ★   OH Clin Surg, 4th edn → pp480, 638

The chest drain has probably become displaced and this would be identified on a review of the chest. 'B' follows 'A' in the 'ABC' of resuscitation and so is the next logical step. A repeat chest X-ray may then be indicated once the patient is stabilized. It is very unlikely for a young patient to require diuresis in trauma resuscitation. This may occasionally be indicated in the situation of pulmonary oedema due to fluid overload. See Figure 15.1.

7. C ★

Compliance is a measure of distensibility of the left ventricle during diastole. Cardiac catheterization or echocardiography can be used to measure left ventricular end-diastolic pressure as a surrogate measure of compliance. Cardiac index is the cardiac output (CO) adjusted to take into account, the size of the patient (cardiac index = CO/body surface area). Left atrial pressure and central venous pressures (CVPs) are indirect measures of preload (filling pressures). Systemic vascular resistance (SVR) reflects the degree of peripheral vasoconstriction and is used as an indirect measurement of afterload. (SVR = Mean arterial pressure (MAP) − CVP/CO) × 80. MAP is calculated by adding a third of the difference between systolic and diastolic pressures to the diastolic pressure.

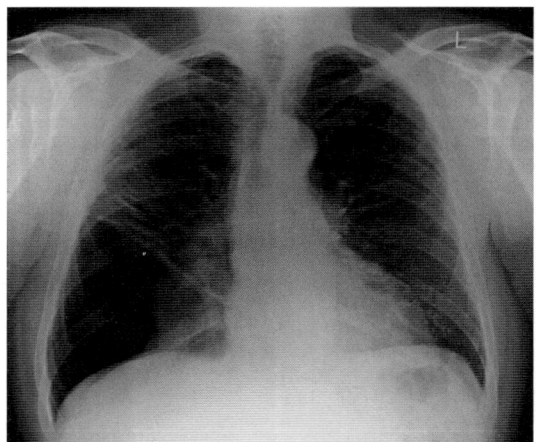

Figure 15.1 A repeat X-ray may be indicated once the patient is stabilized

Reproduced from Gardiner and Borley, *Oxford Specialty Training in Surgery*, 2009, with permission from Oxford University Press.

8. D ★★★   OH Clin Surg, 4th edn → p622

Therapeutic heparinization during bypass surgery is reversed by protamine administration on completion of surgery.

Cardioplegia is the most commonly employed technique for arresting the beating heart during CABG. It is a potassium-rich solution which may be based on blood or crystalloid. It can be delivered warm or cold and is administered directly either into the coronary arteries or coronary sinus vein. Cooling reduces the metabolic demands of the heart. In CABG, blood is derived from the venous side of the circuit by cannulation of inferior vena cava, superior vena cava, or right atrium, passed through the oxygenator and returned to the body by a cannula secured into the ascending aorta. Highest long-term patency rates are achieved with internal mammary artery grafts. Other arterial grafts (e.g. radial artery) have superior long-term patencies compared to vein grafts, which have good early patency (90% at 1 year) but are usually reserved for non-left anterior descending territories. The left internal mammary artery derived from the left subclavian artery is conveniently situated to use as a bypass conduit to the left anterior descending coronary artery. Other commonly employed grafts include reversed long saphenous vein and radial artery. These are anastomosed between the ascending aorta and the diseased coronary artery distal to the stenosis.

9. C ★★   OH Clin Surg, 4th edn → p639

Myasthenia gravis is associated with thymoma in 15% of cases. The diagnostic Tensilon test involves IV injection of a short-acting anticholinesterase, which should result in an increase in muscle power. Thymoma is associated with positive anti-skeletal muscle antibodies.

The anterior mediastinum extends from the thoracic inlet to the line between the sternal angle and the T4–5 intervertebral space. The phrenic nerves are contained in the superior and middle mediastinum. The thymus is found in the anterior mediastinum and is the site for maturation of T cells in early life. See Figure 15.2.

(a)

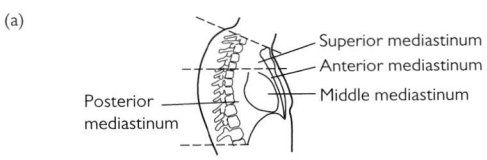

- Superior mediastinum
- Anterior mediastinum
- Middle mediastinum

Posterior mediastinum

(b)

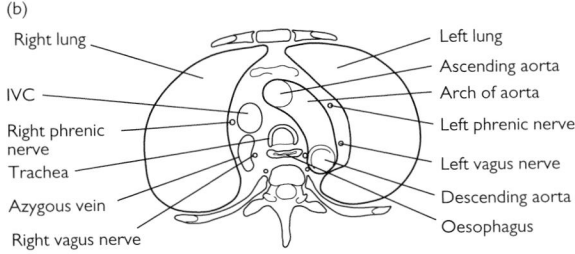

Right lung
IVC
Right phrenic nerve
Trachea
Azygous vein
Right vagus nerve

Left lung
Ascending aorta
Arch of aorta
Left phrenic nerve
Left vagus nerve
Descending aorta
Oesophagus

Figure 15.2 The mediastinum
Reproduced from Chikwe, Cooke, and Weiss, *Oxford Specialist Handbook of Cardiothoracic Surgery*, 2nd edition, 2013, with permission from Oxford University Press.

Extended Matching Questions

1. F ★   OH Clin Surg, 4th edn → p121

Female, hormone replacement therapy or oral contraception, and a recent long-haul flight with associated immobility and therefore venous stasis, are all risk factors for pulmonary embolus.

2. G ★   OH Clin Surg, 4th edn → p628

Shortness of breath, orthopnoea, and paroxysmal nocturnal dyspnoea are all symptoms of heart failure which support the diagnosis of pulmonary oedema.

3. B ★★ OH Clin Surg, 4th edn → p632

A spouse exposed to asbestos at work and bringing the fibres back into the household is a risk factor for mesothelioma.

4. E ★ OH Clin Surg, 4th edn → p636

Primary pneumothorax is idiopathic and is commonly seen in young male smokers of aesthenic build.

5. I ★ OH Clin Surg, 4th edn → p632

This patient has 'red flag' symptoms of bronchial carcinoma and symptoms of upper airway disease. Squamous cell carcinoma commonly affects the large airways and manifests with upper airway obstructive symptoms.

6. I ★★ OH Clin Surg, 4th edn → p628

Following injection of infected material the pulmonary valve may become colonized leading to recurrent pneumonia as infected material embolizes to the lungs. Often more than one valve may be affected, emboli from aortic or mitral valve vegetations in the left heart giving rise to splinter haemorrhages. The clinical picture of subacute bacterial endocarditis may become apparent.

7. K ★★ OH Clin Surg, 4th edn → p628

Retrograde blood flow to the liver due to right ventricular contraction results in pulsatile hepatomegaly and mild jaundice. If the patient also has saphenofemoral incompetence with varicose veins, the pulse will be transmitted in a retrograde fashion resulting in pulsatile reflux in the veins.

8. G ★★ OH Clin Surg, 4th edn → p628

Paravalvular jets of blood bypassing the valve causes the murmur and, in this turbulent blood flow, haemolysis results in a reduction in haemoglobin and a rise in bilirubin.

9. J ★★ OH Clin Surg, 4th edn → p628

Ischaemia can result in the rupture of a papillary muscle, the unsupported mitral valve segment may then prolapse as the left ventricle contracts. Note that this phenomenon is often fatal.

10. B ★★★ OH Clin Surg, 4th edn → p628

Reduced cardiac output due to aortic stenosis is a cause of syncope. The slow rising pulse and systolic murmur confirm the aortic valve's role in this scenario. An aortic murmur may radiate to the carotid arteries. Transthoracic echocardiography is diagnostic. There may be coincidental concomitant vascular disease and unrecognized aortic stenosis increases the risk of vascular surgery.

Chapter 16

Vascular surgery

Oliver Old

As the patient in clinic describes the cramp-like pain that he gets in his calf when he walks, a pain that disappears on resting but which is exacerbated by walking up hills and necessitates him stopping to look in shop windows when out and about, you will be thinking about questioning him for risk factors for vascular disease. Atherosclerosis is a systemic disease. Identification and early treatment of diabetes, hypercholesterolaemia, hypertension, and provision of antiplatelet agents and smoking cessation therapy will confer important cardio- and cerebroprotective benefits.

Acute vascular emergencies requiring an urgent response include the patient with sudden onset, limb-threatening ischaemia; the collapsed patient with a ruptured aortic aneurysm; and the patient in whom haemorrhage or ischaemia comprises part of the picture of complex trauma. Rapid, but thorough examination, appropriate resuscitation, and judicious use of diagnostic imaging will help to underpin urgent management and interventions necessary to obtain the best outcomes for these patients.

Despite increasing reliance on minimally invasive diagnostic modalities including duplex Doppler ultrasound, magnetic resonance angiography, and computed tomography angiography, principles of history taking and good clinical examination remain of paramount importance. Observation to detect nuances of ischaemic trophic changes and skin colour, as well as more overt signs of necrosis, gangrene, and ulceration, complements palpation of pulses, detection of subtle changes in skin temperature, delayed capillary refill, and presence of sensory neuropathy. A positive Buerger's test, with pallor of the foot and venous guttering on leg elevation, and rubor (redness), due to reactive hyperaemia on dependency, may help clinch the diagnosis of critical limb ischaemia when other diagnostic features are equivocal.

Careful distinction between features of arterial insufficiency, venous hypertension, and diabetic neuropathy may help to determine aetiology of a recalcitrant lower limb ulcer and the consequent course of management.

In the UK, vascular surgery has recently become an independent surgical specialty. This chapter will test your understanding of signs and symptoms of vascular disease and will hopefully stimulate your understanding of priorities for investigation and management of the range of conditions comprising this exciting sphere of surgery.

Frank Smith

QUESTIONS

Single Best Answers

1. A 61-year-old man is admitted to the emergency department with sudden onset of a painful, cold, white right leg. His radial pulse rate is 86bpm and its rhythm follows no discernible pattern throughout 30sec of palpation. Abdominal examination is normal. No pulses are palpable in the right leg and ankle Doppler signals are absent. An ECG confirms the arrhythmia but shows no signs of acute ischaemia. Which is the *single* most likely diagnosis? ★

A Abdominal aortic aneurysm

B Aorto-iliac dissection

C Atrial fibrillation

D Deep vein thrombosis

E Myocardial infarction

2. A 70-year-old woman develops a cold, painful, right leg. No pulses are palpable throughout the right leg. She has several risk factors for atherosclerotic disease. A medical student asks how best to differentiate between acute and chronic ischaemia. Which is the *single* most appropriate advice? ★

A History of 40 pack-years of smoking

B History of intermittent claudication

C History of thrombotic stroke

D Presence of femoro-popliteal bypass scar in the left leg

E Presence of foot pulses in the left leg

3. A 65-year-old woman with a 40-pack-year smoking history and type 2 diabetes presents with cramp-like pain in her right calf after walking 500 metres, relieved by rest. Her symptoms are aggravated by walking up steep hills. Which is the *single* most appropriate management? ★★

A Amputation

B Diagnostic angiography

C Endovascular stent

D Modification of risk factors

E Reassure and follow up in 6 months

4. A 55-year-old man who smokes 40 cigarettes per day presents with a history of pain in his left calf after walking 100 metres. The pain goes with rest. He has no symptoms in his thigh or buttock. He has a good volume femoral pulse but no popliteal or pedal pulses are palpable. Neurological examination is normal. He undergoes duplex Doppler ultrasound. Which is the *single* most likely finding of this investigation? ★★★★

A Left common iliac artery occlusion

B Left internal iliac artery stenosis

C Left posterior tibial artery occlusion

D Left profunda femoris artery stenosis

E Left superficial femoral artery occlusion

5. A 69-year-old man is referred to the vascular clinic after an abdominal aortic aneurysm was detected coincidentally on ultrasound examination. The patient is nervous about the diagnosis, has been researching it on the Internet and has several questions. Which *single* statement is correct? ★★

A Abdominal aortic aneurysms are associated with tobacco smoking, hypertension, family history, and diabetes mellitus

B Abdominal aortic aneurysms are considered for treatment by surgical or endovascular repair when they reach a size of ≥5.5cm, in a patient fit for intervention

C Abdominal aortic aneurysms most commonly involve the aorta at the level of the renal arteries and below

D Abdominal aortic aneurysms occur in 10% of the population aged over 65

E Abdominal aortic aneurysm screening is undertaken in the UK using CT scanning

6. A 68-year-old man is referred to the vascular clinic with two recent episodes of transient visual loss in his right eye lasting a few seconds, which he describes as a wave of darkness from top to bottom. He is a lifelong smoker and takes an angiotensin-converting enzyme inhibitor for hypertension, but takes no other medication and is otherwise fit. Duplex Doppler ultrasound of his carotid arteries shows a >70% stenosis at the origin of the right internal carotid artery, and a >90% stenosis of the left internal carotid artery. He is commenced on best medical treatment. Which *single* option is the most appropriate management? ★★★

A Bilateral carotid endarterectomies

B Left carotid endarterectomy

C Reassurance and discharge to GP

D Review in 1 month to monitor visual loss

E Right carotid endarterectomy

7. A 75-year-old woman has a painful non-healing ulcer over the left medial malleolus. It measures 4cm in diameter, with a shallow, superficially infected base, but little evidence of granulation tissue. Despite meticulous nursing care with compression bandaging in the community, the ulcer has shown no sign of improvement over 4 months. She is hypertensive, has angina, chronic obstructive pulmonary disease, and had a deep vein thrombosis in her left leg 10 years ago. She reports no symptoms of intermittent claudication or rest pain. On examination the feet are warm bilaterally, capillary refill time is less than 2sec, both popliteal pulses are palpable but foot pulses are impalpable in both feet. The ankle brachial pressure index is 0.78 on the left and 0.76 on the right. Which *single* option is the most likely underlying cause for her persistent ulceration? ★★

A Chronic lower limb ischaemia

B Diabetic foot disease

C Mixed arterial-venous disease

D Neuropathic ulcer

E Venous insufficiency

8. A 79-year-old man on an inpatient ward becomes acutely short of breath 36h after a right carotid endarterectomy. He has experienced rapidly worsening shortness of breath over the last 4min. His previous medical history includes a transient ischaemic attack 3 weeks ago, myocardial infarction 12 months ago, hypertension, deep vein thrombosis aged 50, and he has been a lifelong smoker. He has a respiratory rate of 45 breaths per minute, oxygen saturation of 89% on air, pulse rate of 120bpm, and blood pressure is 143/78mmHg. He has bruising and swelling around the wound in his neck. Which is the *single* most likely diagnosis? ★★★

A Ipsilateral cerebrovascular accident

B Myocardial infarction

C Pulmonary embolus

D Vagus nerve injury

E Wound haematoma

9. A 48-year-old man with type 1 diabetes and peripheral vascular disease develops an infected ulcer in his right foot. The infection spreads to involve the soft tissues of the foot resulting in necrosis, he develops rigors and his diabetes becomes harder to control with insulin. An amputation is planned and a medical student asks about the procedure and its likely outcome. Which is the *single* most appropriate advice? ★★

A Above-knee amputation is preferred to supracondylar (Gritti–Stokes) amputation for bilateral amputees

B Diabetics are 50 times more likely than non-diabetics to undergo major lower limb amputation

C Likelihood of mobility following below-knee amputation is significantly better than following above-knee amputation

D Postoperative phantom-limb pain is less common in below-knee amputations than above-knee amputations

E Stump healing rates following below-knee amputation are higher than following above-knee amputation

10. A 23-year-old medical student returning from her elective in Australia develops a tender, warm, swollen right calf within 12h of her flight. She smokes five cigarettes daily and takes the oral contraceptive pill. She has no chest pain or shortness of breath. Which *single* investigation is the most appropriate? ★

A Ascending venography

B CT pulmonary angiography

C D dimer

D Duplex ultrasound scan

E VQ scan

11. A 22-year-old woman employed on the butcher's counter at her local supermarket complains that her fingers become white, then blue and cold at work. When she warms her hands under the hot tap they become acutely painful developing a deep red colour. Which is the *single* most appropriate management? ★★★

A Oral prednisolone

B Request transfer from her current job to a different role

C Lumbar sympathectomy

D Oral prostacyclin

E Nifedipine 5mg three times daily increasing to 20mg three times daily

Extended Matching Questions

Vascular symptoms in the legs

For each patient choose the *single* most likely diagnosis from the list of options. Each option may be used once, more than once, or not at all.

A Aorto-iliac arterial disease

B Cellulitis

C Deep vein thrombosis

D Lipodermatosclerosis

E Lymphoedema

F Raynaud's phenomenon

G Scleroderma

H Superficial femoral artery occlusion

I Superficial thrombophlebitis

1. A 58-year-old shopkeeper taking hormone replacement therapy, who has smoked all her working life, develops warm, tender swelling of her calf and thigh at the end of her holiday in Mallorca. She relates this to a wasp sting 3 days earlier. ★★

2. A 75-year-old retired miner who has smoked 30 cigarettes per day for 40 years has cramp-like pain in his calves, thighs, and buttocks which stops him walking after 20 yards on the flat. ★★

3. A 45-year-old woman chef with angular stomatitis has a recent history of dysphagia to solids and fingers with tight skin and trophic nail changes, which go pale then blue on exposure to cold. ★★★★

4. A 52-year-old banker has an acutely tender, warm, reddened varicose vein in his left calf. Three years ago he had an anterior resection for a Duke's B adenocarcinoma of the rectum. ★★

5. A 43-year-old office worker, who has had a swollen left leg since her early teens, has aching in the calf at rest and has developed a 4cm shallow ulcer, with an erythematous base, above her lateral malleolus. ★★★

Amputations

For each patient choose the *single* most appropriate amputation from the list of options. Each option may be used once, more than once, or not at all.

A Above-knee

B Below-knee

C Digital

D Gritti–Stokes (supracondylar)

E Hip disarticulation

F Ray

G Symes

H Through-knee

I Transmetatarsal

6. A 52-year-old type 1 diabetic man has wet gangrene of the 2nd and 3rd toes and infection tracking back into the webspaces. Posterior tibial and dorsalis pedis pulses are palpable. ★★

7. A 47-year-old woman has noticed a brown pigmented lesion beneath the toenail on her left hallux. Excision of the toenail and biopsy confirms the presence of a subungual melanoma. ★★

8. A 68-year-old insulin-dependent diabetic man who smokes 30 cigarettes a day has a necrotic heel ulcer which has eroded into the calcaneum. His temperature is 38.2°C and his blood sugar is 18mmol/L (higher than normal) on his usual insulin dose. X-rays confirm extensive osteomyelitis of the calcaneum. Magnetic resonance angiography demonstrates a patent popliteal artery, but no patent calf or pedal vessels. ★★★

9. A 55-year-old wheelchair-dependent woman with multiple sclerosis and lower limb paralysis has extensive suppurating circumferential ulceration around the gaiter area of her left leg due to dependent oedema. This has proved recalcitrant to all treatment. She relies on her husband to transfer her from the chair to her bed. She has suffered from episodes of systemic sepsis and the smell of the ulcer is causing her great distress. She requests amputation, a request which is supported by her family. ★★★★

10. A 27-year-old motorcyclist has suffered from comminuted distal femoral and open tibial fractures after being involved in a road traffic collision in which his lower leg was run over by a lorry. Neurological examination confirms that he has no sensation or movement from the level of the knee distally. Surgical debridement reveals extensive muscle necrosis in all calf muscle compartments. He has myoglobinuria and a serum creatinine of 190μmol/L. ★★★★

ANSWERS

Single Best Answers

1. **C** ★   OH Clin Surg, 4th edn → p642

The presentation is that of an embolic episode with occluded flow to the femoral artery. Emboli account for 30% of acute limb ischaemia. Eighty per cent of emboli have a cardiac cause (e.g. atrial fibrillation, myocardial infarction, ventricular aneurysm); 10% result from proximal peripheral arterial aneurysms (including aortic aneurysms). Rarer causes of acute leg ischaemia include aorto-iliac dissection, trauma, iatrogenic injury, intra-arterial drug use. The finding of an irregular pulse suggests this as the likely cause in this patient. No aneurysm was palpable on abdominal examination and aorto-iliac dissection is less likely. Deep vein thrombosis is an unlikely cause of acute lower limb arterial ischaemia, but this may occur rarely when a deep vein thrombosis embolizes with resulting embolus passing through a patent foramen ovale defect in the heart, allowing passage of the embolus from venous to arterial systems. This is termed a paradoxical embolus. A patent foramen ovale may occur in 27–35% of the normal population and in patients with a patent foramen ovale, major pulmonary embolus may be accompanied by peripheral arterial embolism in up to 15% of cases.

→ Konstantinides S, Geibel A, Kasper W, et al. Patent foramen ovale is an important predictor of adverse outcome in patients with major pulmonary embolism. *Circulation* 1998; 97:1946–51.

2. **E** ★   OH Clin Surg, 4th edn → p647

Clinical features indicating atherosclerotic disease, e.g. risk factors for atherosclerosis (smoking, hypercholesterolaemia, hypertension), history of peripheral arterial disease, coronary artery disease, or cerebrovascular disease, would suggest that chronic lower limb ischaemia is likely. However, the presence of good contralateral pulses in a patient presenting with absent pulses in one lower limb strongly suggests acute lower limb ischaemia.

3. **D** ★★   OH Clin Surg, 4th edn → p647

Intermittent claudication is twice as common in males as females. Risk factors include hypertension, hypercholesterolaemia, diabetes mellitus, smoking, and positive family history. All patients with intermittent claudication should undergo assessment of risk factors. Patients should be advised to stop smoking, and to take regular exercise. Treatment with aspirin and statins, and control of blood pressure with angiotensin-converting enzyme inhibitors such as ramipril, has been shown to reduce risk of mortality from myocardial infarction and stroke. Good blood glucose control should reduce the incidence of diabetic complications. Approximately one-third of patients with intermittent claudication improve, one-third remain stable, and one-third deteriorate, but only 4% require intervention and in only 1% is amputation eventually necessary. Note that diabetic patients may have calcified incompressible arteries and assessment of the degree of ischaemia by measurement of ankle brachial pressure indices may therefore be unreliable.

→ Norgren L, Hiatt WR, Dormandy JA, et al.; TASC II Working Group. Inter-Society Consensus for the Management of Peripheral Arterial Disease (TASC II). *J Vasc Surg* 2007; 45(Suppl S):S5–67.

4. E ★★★★   OH Clin Surg, 4th edn → p647

An occlusion is a complete blockage of an artery whereas a stenosis implies narrowing of the vessel. Calf claudication is most commonly caused by superficial femoral arterial disease. Absent popliteal and pedal pulses suggest that significant symptomatic arterial disease exists proximal to the level of the popliteal artery. If the femoral pulse is of good volume, common iliac artery occlusion is unlikely. Disease of the internal iliac artery may cause buttock claudication and/or impotence (Leriche's syndrome). Common iliac or external iliac disease may cause thigh claudication, in addition to calf claudication. Profunda femoris disease often contributes to thigh and calf claudication, but is unlikely to cause calf claudication in isolation.

5. B ★★   OH Clin Surg, 4th edn → p647

Abdominal aortic aneurysms are associated with hypertension, smoking, family history, but not with diabetes mellitus. Other rarer causes include infective causes ('mycotic') and connective tissue disorders. The UK Small Aneurysm Trial suggested that intervention for abdominal aortic aneurysms should be undertaken when the aneurysm reaches a threshold diameter of 5.5cm. A national screening programme for aortic aneurysms is being implemented in the UK, in which ultrasound detection is the screening modality of choice. CT would not be an appropriate screening tool due to high radiation dose and cost. Abdominal aortic aneurysms occur in 5% of males over 65 (they are approximately nine times commoner in men than in women). Ninety-five per cent of abdominal aortic aneurysms are infrarenal; 15% extend into the common iliac arteries.

→ The UK Small Aneurysm Trial Participants. Mortality results for randomised controlled trial of early elective surgery or ultrasonographic surveillance for small abdominal aortic aneurysms. *Lancet* 1998; 352(9141):1649–55.

6. E ★★★   OH Clin Surg, 4th edn → pp652, 654

The patient is describing amaurosis fugax, transient monocular visual loss, which represents a transient ischaemic attack in the central retinal artery, in the carotid territory on the ipsilateral (right) side. Symptomatic patients with >70% stenosis should be offered carotid endarterectomy on the affected side which, in addition to best medical treatment, should reduce the risk of stroke to 3–5%. Surgery should be undertaken as soon as possible since the risk of stroke is greatest in the first month following a transient ischaemic attack. Benefits of surgery for asymptomatic patients are less, so endarterectomy is not indicated for the contralateral (left) side at this time, in this case. There is no benefit from endarterectomy if the artery is completely occluded. Best medical therapy should be commenced irrespective of surgery: this reduces the risk of stroke in the 12 months following TIA to approximately 18%.

→ Cina CS, Clase CM, Haynes RB. Carotid endarterectomy for symptomatic carotid stenosis. *Cochrane Database Syst Rev* 2000; 2:CD001081.

7. C ★★   OH Clin Surg, 4th edn → p658

The ulcer is located in the gaiter area of the leg, a characteristic site for venous ulcers. A history of deep venous thrombosis may have rendered the deep veins incompetent, predisposing to venous hypertension, skin changes, and ulceration (post-phlebitic syndrome).

However, failure to heal despite treatment with compression bandaging suggests that there may also be underlying arterial insufficiency, confirmed by reduced ankle brachial pressure indices.

Diabetic foot disease affects the foot as a result of the interdependent triad of neuropathy, ischaemia, and infection. This ulcer is not characteristic of diabetic foot disease and is painful, so neuropathy is unlikely to be a causative factor.

8. E ★★★   OH Clin Surg, 4th edn → pp666, 668

A sudden deterioration implies an acute event. Given the history of recent carotid endarterectomy with neck swelling, a wound haematoma compromising the airway must be suspected. This may occur due to bleeding at the site of the arteriotomy, carotid patch blow out, or delayed wound bleeding, which may be arterial or venous in origin. This can rapidly obstruct the airway and prove fatal unless the swelling is relieved— these patients need immediate re-opening of the neck incision, on the ward if necessary, to drain the haematoma, and to apply pressure to the bleeding point, with urgent transfer to theatre. Cerebrovascular accident would usually present with neurological signs. Myocardial infarction is an acknowledged complication of endarterectomy but rarely presents with acute dyspnoea alone. Pulmonary embolus is a rare complication of endarterectomy and the time course following surgery is usually longer. A vagus nerve injury may cause dyspnoea due to adduction of the ipsilateral vocal cord but this would usually be apparent in the immediate recovery period following surgery.

9. C ★★   OH Clin Surg, 4th edn → p658

For bilateral amputees, preservation of limb length is important for balance, especially if they are likely to be confined to a wheelchair. The Gritti–Stokes amputation preserves more of the femur than an above-knee amputation. Diabetics are 15 times more likely to require amputation than non-diabetics. Stump healing rates are related to level of amputation and adequacy of blood supply, which is generally better proximally in the limb. There is no evidence to suggest phantom-limb pain occurs less frequently in below-knee amputations.

10. D ★   OH Clin Surg, 4th edn → p668

This student has clinical features suggestive of a deep vein thrombosis. This may be demonstrated by ascending venography, but this requires contrast injection and has been superseded by duplex ultrasound scanning which is sensitive and non-invasive. CT pulmonary angiography is the modality of choice for rapid and sensitive investigation for suspected pulmonary embolus. It has now largely replaced ventilation perfusion (VQ) scans for investigation of pulmonary embolism. D dimers are a sensitive test for deep vein thrombosis but are usually employed as part of a thrombotic screen. The most sensitive, specific, and appropriate investigation in this case is duplex ultrasound of the leg which will demonstrate occlusive thrombus and blood flow disturbances caused by clot.

11. B ★★★   OH Clin Surg, 4th edn → p664

This woman is exhibiting Raynaud's phenomenon on exposure of her hands to a cold stimulus. This occurs nine times more commonly in females and characteristically affects young women. The redness of her hands on warming is caused by reactive hyperaemia, not a reperfusion injury, which is often accompanied by pain and paraesthesia. Initial management should be based around conservative measures including avoidance of cold stimuli, stopping smoking, and wearing gloves where feasible. If this fails, second-line therapy involves treatment with calcium channel blockers, such as nifedipine, in the doses described (E). In debilitating digital vasospasm resistant to other treatments, IV infusions of prostacyclin, titrated against body mass and side effects, may provide respite. Lumbar chemical sympathectomy is occasionally employed to improve cutaneous blood flow and to relieve rest pain in critical leg ischaemia, but has no role here. Steroids are not an appropriate treatment.

Extended Matching Questions

1. C ★★   OH Clin Surg, 4th edn → p668

This lady has clinical features suggestive of deep vein thrombosis. Risk factors include use of hormonal medications, smoking, and dehydration. Insect bites may be associated with cellulitis and localized oedematous reactions but the time scale suggests this is not a likely causative factor.

2. A ★★   OH Clin Surg, 4th edn → p647

This man's leg symptoms are characteristic of atherosclerotic occlusive arterial disease affecting the aorta and/or iliac arteries.

3. G ★★★★   OH Clin Surg, 4th edn → p664

This woman has a history suggestive of scleroderma, in association with other symptoms including oesophageal dysmotility, which may form part of the CREST syndrome (Calcinosis, Raynaud's phenomenon, oEsophageal dysmotility, Sclerodactyly, Telangiectasia). This syndrome forms part of the spectrum of connective tissue diseases which are associated with Raynaud's phenomenon.

4. I ★★   OH Clin Surg, 4th edn → p666

This man has a tender inflamed varicosity likely to be due to superficial thrombophlebitis. This may be idiopathic but may also occur in association with a variety of other conditions including infection, pregnancy, IV cannulation, and malignancies. Investigations in this case should aim to exclude recurrent carcinoma in addition to establishing the diagnosis of superficial thrombophlebitis, which can be done with ultrasound.

5. E ★★★   OH Clin Surg, 4th edn → p656

This lady has a history suggestive of congenital unilateral lymphoedema (Milroy's disease), associated with hypoplasia of the lymphatic trunks. Long-term lymphoedema predisposes to skin changes including leg ulcers, fungal infections, and increased risk of cellulitis. The mainstay of conservative management is treatment with compression and expectant management of superficial skin infections with early antibiotic treatment. Lymphoscintigraphy may be helpful in confirming the diagnosis.

6. F ★★   OH Clin Surg, 4th edn → p662

The appropriate amputation here is a ray amputation which is undertaken to amputate the necrotic toes and to treat localized sepsis tracking back into the foot. The blood supply should be adequate to ensure healing and full debridement of all necrotic tissue should be undertaken. The wound will either be left open to heal by secondary intention or closed loosely over a drain.

7. C ★★   OH Clin Surg, 4th edn → p662

Digital amputation will be undertaken in this case to excise the melanoma. Histopathological staging will be assessed by measuring the Breslow thickness. If there is spread to nodes, block node dissection may also be indicated.

8. B ★★★ OH Clin Surg, 4th edn → p662

This patient has a bone infection which will not be cleared by antibiotic treatment. Angiography suggests extensive underlying arterial disease, not amenable to arterial reconstruction, so local procedures to debride infected tissues will be unlikely to heal. Provided that the blood supply is adequate to the level of the knee, a below-knee amputation employing either long posterior flap or skew flap technique will be likely to heal and will provide the best chance of subsequent mobility with a prosthetic limb.

9. D ★★★★ OH Clin Surg, 4th edn → p662

This patient is not weightbearing on her legs, nor able to use them to transfer. She is suffering from significant debility from her dependent leg ulcer and in the face of failed treatments to get the ulcer to heal, her request for amputation is reasonable. A Gritti–Stokes amputation will provide her with the greatest length of limb to aid balancing in her wheelchair. Preservation of the knee will confer no advantage if she is unable to use this joint.

10. A ★★★★ OH Clin Surg, 4th edn → p662

This patient has a flail limb with systemic debility in the form of acute renal impairment caused by extensive muscle necrosis. Above-knee amputation whilst accompanied by significant psychological and physical morbidity is the procedure most likely to allow early recovery and to permit eventual mobilization with a prosthesis.

Chapter 17

Surgery in tropical diseases

Simon Fisher and Serena Ledwidge

Whether you exercise a desire to experience surgery abroad during your student elective or whether you want to take the opportunity to enhance your career aspirations in far-flung regions, knowledge of common surgical presentations of tropical disease is a prerequisite. Moreover, with the ability conferred by modern jet travel to translocate to almost any area of the globe within 48h, you may well encounter these conditions in your local general hospital clinic or emergency department, in visitors to the country or in travellers returning home from foreign excursions.

This chapter tests you on your knowledge of presentations, investigations, and management of diseases such as malaria, schistosomiasis, amoebiasis, and filariasis, conditions native to a variety of geographical locations. Some diseases such as hydatid still remain endemic in regions closer to the UK.

A sound understanding of parasitic life cycles, modes of exposure to, and manifestations of infection, and principles of treatment, will help you to diagnose and manage these conditions whether they are encountered unexpectedly, or prevalent in your geographical location.

Frank Smith

QUESTIONS

Single Best Answers

1. A 25-year-old man has been in a malaria-endemic region for 3 days. He has had diarrhoea for 36h but has no other symptoms. Pulse is 92bpm, temperature is 38.2°C. Which is the *single* most appropriate management? ★★★★

A Administer loperamide and review again in 24h

B Administer rehydration salts and review again in 24h

C Administer rehydration salts and review again in 48h

D Take blood for FBC and a blood film

E Take blood for U&E

2. A 15-year-old girl returns from 2 weeks in a typhoid-endemic region. She has a 4-day history of abdominal pain and foul green-yellow diarrhoea. Temperature is 38°C. Which is the *single* most appropriate diagnostic test? ★★★★

A Blood film

B Blood serology

C FBC

D Plain abdominal X-ray

E Stool microscopy

3. A 15-year-old girl returns from 2 weeks in a typhoid-endemic region. She has a 4-day history of abdominal pain and foul green-yellow diarrhoea. Temperature is 38.7 °C. On examination she has abdominal guarding, rebound tenderness, and absent bowel sounds. Which is the *single* most appropriate next step? ★★★

A CT scan abdomen/pelvis

B Exploratory laparotomy

C Rigid or flexible sigmoidoscopy

D Stool culture with selective enrichment media

E Take blood for serology

4. A 42-year-old man returned yesterday from a 3-week trip in the tropics. He has had night sweats and rigors for 2 days and episodic bloody diarrhoea for 9 days. His abdomen is tender in the right upper quadrant with hepatomegaly. His temperature is 37.9°C, pulse is 93bpm. Which is the *single* most appropriate initial investigation? ★★★★

A Abdominal ultrasound scan

B Blood film

C FBC

D LFTs

E Stool microscopy and culture

5. A 35-year-old woman returned yesterday from the Middle East. For 4 days she has had pain on passing urine, and mentions she has been passing water more than once per hour. She has noticed blood in her urine. Which is the *single* most appropriate investigation? ★★★★

A CT scan kidneys/ureter/bladder

B Cystoscopy and bladder biopsy

C Microscopy of early morning urine

D Ultrasound scan kidneys/ureter/bladder

E Urine dipstick for leucocytes and nitrites

6. A 52-year-old man who owns a sheep farm in Wales has a 6-month history of vague abdominal discomfort but is otherwise well. An abdominal ultrasound scan is performed and a liver cyst is found. Which is the *single* most appropriate diagnostic test? ★★★★

A Casoni's test for serum antigen

B CT scan abdomen/pelvis

C ERCP

D Indirect haemagglutination tests

E Ultrasound-guided cyst aspiration

ANSWERS

Single Best Answers

1. D ★★★★ OH Clin Surg, 4th edn → p710

In areas where dengue or malaria occurs, a fever lasting more than a day even with focal symptoms such as diarrhoea, requires a FBC and blood film.

2. B ★★★★ OH Clin Surg, 4th edn → p704

Typhoid affects older children and young adults with an incubation period of 10–14 days. Onset is gradual and symptoms include high fever, abdominal pain, and pea-soup diarrhoea. Diagnostic tests are serology (Widal test) or stool culture with selective enrichment media (MacConkey or DCA agar).

3. B ★★★ OH Clin Surg, 4th edn → p704

She is peritonitic suggesting intra-abdominal perforation. Complications of typhoid fever include cholecystitis with perforation and intestinal perforation along the antimesenteric border of the ileum at the site of Peyer's patches. The management of intestinal perforation is laparotomy with lavage and closure of the perforation plus IV chloramphenicol. Cholecystitis with perforation might be managed laparoscopically or open with lavage and cholecystectomy plus IV chloramphenicol.

4. A ★★★★ OH Clin Surg, 4th edn → p706

This man has symptoms suggesting hepatic amoebiasis. Abdominal ultrasound scan will allow assessment of the liver for amoebic liver abscess which is a complication of amoebic hepatitis. It may also allow aspiration of pus for diagnosis and treatment. Microscopy and culture of fresh stool may reveal amoebae, but in this case drainage of potential liver abscess would take precedence.

Blood film would be useful for diagnosing malaria. It is prudent in the pyrexial patient returned from the tropics but this clinical scenario puts hepatic amoebiasis ahead of malaria as a differential.

FBC and LFTs will not be diagnostic, though may be abnormal.

5. C ★★★★ OH Clin Surg, 4th edn → p712

Schistosomiasis is endemic in many parts of North Africa, the Middle East, and South-East Asia. Bladder worms can produce inflammation of mucosa and slough leading to dysuria, frequency, and haematuria. Microscopy of early morning urine or a faecal specimen can demonstrate the presence of living eggs. This would be first line in preference to cystoscopy and bladder biopsy which could also provide confirmation of infection.

6. D ★★★★   OH Clin Surg, 4th edn → p716

It is important to consider the diagnosis of a hydatid cyst in this man as hydatid disease is not restricted to the tropics. Infections are well documented in certain areas of Wales and the Western Isles of Scotland. The most accurate diagnostic test is the indirect haemagglutination test. Casoni's test for serum antigen is positive in 80% but gives many false positives. CT scan may be used to localize cysts. ERCP may demonstrate connections with or compression of the bile duct—obstructive jaundice may be found on presentation. Ultrasound-guided cyst aspiration is an option for management but not first line for diagnosis. This is because rupture of a cyst into the peritoneal cavity causes peritonitis and shock. Cyst fluid entering the circulation causes a severe allergic reaction with urticaria and eosinophilia.

Index

Note: Answers to questions appear in *italics*